Sexual Health in Drug and Alcohol Treatment

Doug Braun-Harvey received his master's degree in counseling from National University in 1982. He has been a Licensed Marriage and Family Therapist since 1982 and a Certified Group Psychotherapist since 1994. He founded the Sexual Dependency Institute of San Diego in 1993 to provide outpatient treatment for men with out of control sexual behavior (OCSB). Mr. Braun-Harvey presents nationally and internationally on issues of sexual health, OCSB, and group psychotherapy. He is lecturing faculty in the Masters of Counseling Program at San Diego State University. From 2002 to 2005, he was a consultant to Stepping Stone of San Diego, a residential drug and alcohol treatment center, where he developed and supervised the nation's first sexual behavior relapse prevention program. This pioneering program improved addiction treatment outcomes through a psycho-educational program linking relapse-prevention strategies with principles of sexual health. Currently Mr. Braun-Harvey is in private practice in Mission Valley, San Diego, and is located on the web at www.sexualdependency.com.

Sexual Health in Drug and Alcohol Treatment

Group Facilitator's Manual

DOUGLAS BRAUN-HARVEY, MFT, CGP

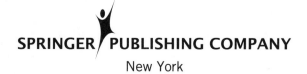

SPRINGER PUBLISHING COMPANY

New York

Springer Publishing Company, LLC
11 West 42nd Street
New York, NY 10036
www.springerpub.com

Acquisitions Editor: Jennifer Perillo
Project Manager: Mark Frazier
Cover Designer: TG Design
Composition: Apex CoVantage, LLC
Ebook ISBN: 978-08261-2016-8

09 10 11 12 13 / 5 4 3 2 1

The author and the publisher of this Work have made every effort to use sources believed to be reliable to provide information that is accurate and compatible with the standards generally accepted at the time of publication. Because medical science is continually advancing, our knowledge base continues to expand. Therefore, as new information becomes available, changes in procedures become necessary. We recommend that the reader always consult current research and specific institutional policies before performing any clinical procedure. The author and publisher shall not be liable for any special, consequential, or exemplary damages resulting, in whole or in part, from the readers' use of, or reliance on, the information contained in this book. The publisher has no responsibility for the persistence or accuracy of URLs for external or third-party Internet Web sites referred to in this publication and does not guarantee that any content on such Web sites is, or will remain, accurate or appropriate.

Library of Congress Cataloging-in-Publication Data

Braun-Harvey, Douglas.
  Sexual health in drug and alcohol treatment : group facilitator's
manual / Douglas Braun-Harvey.
    p. cm.
  Includes bibliographical references and index.
  ISBN 978-0-8261-2015-1 (alk. paper)—ISBN 978-0-8261-2016-8 (ebook)
  1. Drug addiction—Treatment. 2. Alcoholism—Treatment. 3. Sex. I. Title.
  RC564.B717   2009
  616.86'06—dc22   2009026691

Printed in the United States of America by Hamilton Printing.

To Al, my singular sensation and unexpected rainbow

Contents

In the past, substance-abuse treatment counselors focused only on the client's addiction and assumed that other issues would either resolve themselves through recovery or be dealt with by another helping professional at a later time. Over time, with additional research and increased clinical experience, treatment providers began to note the need for comprehensive, integrated services. Many treatment providers today follow the National Institute of Drug Abuse (NIDA) guidelines that state that drug addiction is a complex disorder that can involve virtually every aspect of an individual's functioning. The guidelines recommend that programs provide a combination of therapies and other services to meet the individual needs of each patient. However, even in these contemporary guidelines, the issue of sexuality is not mentioned.

The current neglect of sexuality as a core issue in addiction recovery reflects an experience I had in 1982. I still have a vivid memory of a presentation I gave at a national conference in Washington, D.C. The title of my paper was "Sex and Violence: The Unmentionables in Addiction Treatment." The responses from the attendees ranged from discomfort to anger. Many told me that their clients would relapse if these topics were discussed and that their clients were "not ready" for this work. I tried to explain that clients were at risk of relapse if we did *not* discuss these issues. Later I realized that it was the addiction professionals, not the clients, who were not ready.

In this new evidence-based curriculum, *Sexual Health for Drug and Alcohol Treatment,* Doug Braun-Harvey challenges our attitudes and beliefs as well as our traditional ways of providing treatment. He challenges us to "get ready" and he provides a way to do it. This material on sexual health can help to provide a missing piece for many recovering addicts.

Recovery means more than the elimination of one's drug of choice, either through harm reduction or abstinence. Recovery is also about what is added or gained in one's life. To me, recovery means wholeness. It means having one's inner self (thoughts, feelings, values, and beliefs) *connected and congruent* with one's outer self (behavior and relationships). Developing sexual health in recovery is essential to becoming an integrated, whole person.

In a world in which sex is emphasized so much, in which alcohol and drugs are associated with sexual experiences, and in which the meaning of love is so bewildering to so many, Doug Braun-Harvey stands out as a pioneer in guiding the addiction-treatment field toward sexual health.

Stephanie S. Covington, PhD, LCSW

Acknowledgments

Countless sexual health conversations are reflected in this book. I am humbled by the generosity and enthusiasm of those who have contributed their resources, vision, hope, wisdom, measurement, opinion, criticism, and warm shoulder throughout the last 8 years. Sexual health is an act of collective connection.

In 2001 Cheryl Houk, the former Executive Director of Stepping Stone of San Diego, asked me for help. She was "tired of people dying" because her treatment program was failing to help those with what we have now come to call high sex/drug-linked behavior. Her belief that we can do better has been my centering mantra. The Board of Directors of Stepping Stone allowed Cheryl to explore her vision. We began a volunteer collaboration to change the way sexuality was addressed at Stepping Stone. Cheryl and I were determined to begin saving lives.

It was Cheryl who initiated a conversation with The California Endowment, which lead to the grant to develop sexual health as a means of improving treatment. Greg Hall and Stacy Amodio from The California Endowment were invaluable in fostering and overseeing the 3-year grant. Marc d'Hondt, who unwaveringly believed in this project since its inception, remains a steadfast sexual health advocate at Stepping Stone. Maridia Harrington provided way too much laughter and joy during the many hours in my kitchen going about the work of writing the grant and sowing the seeds for the original concepts in this book.

I remain deeply grateful and indebted to the Stepping Stone staff and volunteers who leapt into a void and trusted the idea that becoming a sex-positive treatment center would help women and men recover. Their hard work, dedication, and inspiration are on every page.

This book reflects the enthusiasm and pride of the hundreds of Stepping Stone clients who completed the sexual health in recovery curriculum. Without their courage to change and daring to be different this book would be yet another wish in the minds of countless treatment providers frustrated by yet another addict "taken out by sex".

In this era of evidence-based treatment a researcher and evaluator with experience, intelligence, and rigorous standards is an important sexual health ally. I was fortunate to find all three in my collaboration with Jim Zians. Jim expertly guided the evolution of this project from clinical concept to funded grant to measurable intervention. He established protocols for Stepping Stone to assess and measure their essential evidence-based outcomes. Thank you Jim for teaching me: "If I can't measure it then it can't be in the curriculum." San Diego social science researchers Linda Lloyd, Tom Patterson, and Tom Smith contributed time and wisdom to the internal review process. The publications of many sexologists, addictionologists, psychotherapists, and stages of change researchers have been essential primary sources of sexual health conversations. I found hope and inspiration in their ideas and science.

Beginning in December 2003 Joe Dintino and Nancy Busch began leading each new curricula and during the proceeding months improving on them each step of the way. They worked hand in hand with me to correct what did not work, confirm what was effective, and assist with strategic changes. It is a rare opportunity to experience this kind of teamwork, trust, and creativity. They were the right people at the right time. When Espen Correll joined the team he brought with him advanced training in human sexuality. He enthusiastically bridged sexual health education among addiction treatment professionals. He got San Diego treatment centers clamoring for sexual heath. John De Miranda, the current CEO of Stepping Stone, is a tireless advocate for improving drug treatment. He knows first hand the benefits of the sexual health program at Stepping Stone and envisions sexual health in recovery as an important contribution for improving treatment outcomes across the nation.

Sexual health conversations with respected and trusted professional colleagues are essential. Members of The Society for the Scientific Study of Sexuality [SSSS]; Southeast Conference on Addictive Disorders [SECAD]; The National Association of Lesbian and Gay Addiction Professionals [NALGAP]; American Association of Sex Educators, Counselors, and Therapists [AASECT]; The Society for the Advancement of Sexual Health [SASH]; The Hazelden Graduate School of Addiction Studies; and The American Group Psychotherapy Association [AGPA] have listened, advised, and confirmed my belief in sexual health becoming an ally with drug and alcohol treatment. Many of these organizations invited Stepping Stone, Jim Zians, and myself to present workshops, trainings, and forums to report early findings and to discuss sexual health as a clinical intervention for improving treatment outcomes and increasing client retention.

I have worked with a diverse spectrum of sexual health allies from around the country. They include Kip Castner, Lori Jones, Carol Crump, Chuck Stonecipher, James Campbell, The Chadwick Center for Children & Families, Heidi Aiem, Steve Bolda, Kenny Goldgerg, Peter Taylor, and David Wohlsifer. Each from disparate professions yet all possessing a vision for sexual health as an ally for improving the lives of the people they serve.

Sexual health is all about the details. I have been privileged with particular gifts of wisdom from many people. Eli Coleman, Stephanie Covington, and Chris Kraft's 2003 curriculum draft peer review in Minneapolis was a turning point in conceptualization, content, and construct validity. Their expert criticism provided invaluable direction, mentoring, and encouragement on that September day and every day since. They are my sex/drug-link advisors. Corrine Casanova contributed early editorial expertise to the curriculum and was a welcome ally and advocate for this book to find a wider audience. George Marcelle provided timely nudging for me to find a publisher. Deanne Gruenberg (Dee Dee) and her husband, Harry, provided book-selling business expertise and matchmaking with Springer Publishing. Dee Dee is a determined advocate for sexual heath.

Sexual health thrives among friends and family. Friends and respected colleagues G. Michael Scott and Ron Robertson were early contributors to the spirituality lesson. Writer Rebecca Cutter is not only a dear friend but also an invaluable mentor in the writing process. Thank you to my many friends at the Special Interest Group for Gay, Lesbian, Bisexual, and Transgender concerns at the American Group Psychotherapy Association. They are my allies in bridging sexual health and group work. With my colleague Michael Vigorito, I have been fortunate to have traversed from being sexual health mentor to collaborator. Peter Wayson, Paul Sussman, Dan Offner, Al Killen-Harvey, David Garmon, G. Michael Scott, and Dan Bjierke comprise a 15-year continuous monthly peer supervision group. Our mutual commitment to looking at ourselves to better the lives of our clients is cherished good fortune. These fine men have witnessed every step of this voyage. Gay Parnell and Rick Avery know all too well my personal and professional writing journey. Listening was their best medicine.

Over many years my sister and best friend Charlotte Braun has laughed with me across the country, lovingly attending many of my conference workshops. Picturing her in 2003 sitting among the Minneapolis attendees at the first presentation of this curriculum is a cherished memory. I am blessed by her support and belief in my work as a sexual health advocate. I owe a debt of thanks to my niece Amy Peterson. She generously shares her hilarious sexual health conversations, sometimes by cell or text, moments after the hilarity. She is a beloved connection for great sexual health stories. My niece Ashley Braun is my tutor for social networking culture. I can humbly be very old with her and she is kind and caring.

My editor Jennifer Perillo has from day one understood the importance of sexual health and has guided the shape of this book with kind and firm enthusiasm. She has been the necessary voice of the outsider calling me to be clear, precise, and well organized.

Finally, to my husband, Al. I love you will all my heart. You have spent way too many weekends taking care of the life of our home, family, and friends while I gaze into my laptop. I could have never completed this book without you. Your support and generous heart is a daily gift of love. You have been my resident sexual health expert since 1987. How convenient!

Proceeds from the sale of this book will be donated to Stepping Stone of San Diego (steppingstonesd.org) and to the Douglas Braun-Harvey Fund for the Program in Human Sexuality in the Department of Family Medicine and Community Health at the University of Minnesota (http://www.fm.umn.edu/phs/phsgift/home.html).

The Creation of the *Sexual Health in Drug and Alcohol Treatment* Curriculum

FROM ABSTINENCE TO RELAPSE

Numerous experts and research studies have demonstrated that addicts in recovery are extremely susceptible to relapse. "Lapse, defined as re-use of alcohol or drugs at least once following treatment, occurs in at least 50% of those who complete treatment. . . . Relapse, defined as return to excessive or problematic use . . . [occurs] in approximately 20–30% of those who complete formal care in the prior year" (McLellan, 2007). Others agree: "There is now broad agreement in the clinical research community that addiction is best characterized by a chronic disease that for most people includes occasional relapses" (Lesher, 2003, p. 194). "Relapse rates for addictive diseases do not differ significantly from rates for other chronic diseases. Relapse rates for addictive diseases range from 50 percent for resumption of heavy use to 90 percent for a brief lapse" (Gordon, 2003, p. 6).

For addiction professionals, the question is: *Why* are addicts so prone to relapse? Scientific research is changing our understanding of the nature of addiction. New studies in brain imaging provide compelling visual data revealing changes in the brain circuitry of addicts (Childress et al., 1999; Volkow et al., 1999). Thus, we now understand addiction as a combination of changes in the addicted person's brain structure and chemistry as well as his or her behavior and social circumstances (Lesher, 2003).

Such findings can increase our compassion for the persistent pattern of relapse among addicts in recovery, and help us understand that many addicts require multiple treatments before they achieve a stable abstinence. Normalizing drug and alcohol relapse as a predictable course in the treatment of a chronic disease (similar to relapses often encountered in the treatment of chronic illnesses like asthma, heart disease, obesity, and diabetes) has allowed for a more reasoned discussion among drug treatment professionals regarding the role of relapse and for significant changes in treatment approaches.

FROM RELAPSE TO TREATMENT

Relapse during or following treatment has long been a source of consternation and frustration for addicts, their families, and those who treat them. The ideal of successful treatment is to maintain abstinence for the rest of the addict's life, yet few treatment programs meet this goal.

In the early 1990s, experts and researchers began comparing outcomes of varying addiction treatments in the hopes of improving relapse prevention. They wanted to discover if any particular treatment was statistically significantly superior to the others. One of the most widely cited research studies from this period was a multi-site alcohol treatment clinical trial matching alcohol treatments to client heterogeneity called Project MATCH. This 8-year study, conducted by the National Institute on Alcohol Abuse and Alcoholism (NIAAA), analyzed alcohol treatment outcomes among three groups, each utilizing a different treatment paradigm: 12-step facilitation (based on the principles of Alcoholics Anonymous), cognitive-behavioral therapy (based on social learning theory), or motivational enhancement therapy (based on motivational psychology). Participants in each group were matched to a particular treatment based on their characteristics, including severity of alcohol use, cognitive impairment, gender, motivational readiness to change, social support for drinking versus abstinence, and other factors (Project MATCH Research Group, 1993).

Overall, the findings of Project MATCH confirmed 1 hypothetical match and did not confirm 10 others, leading researches to the conclude that treatment outcomes were not correlated with patient-treatment matching. (National Institute on Alcohol Abuse and Alcoholism [NIAAA], 1996). Numerous follow-up studies have supported this initial data. Specific treatments targeted and matched with specific populations were no longer the singular focus of relapse prevention. A new direction beckoned.

FROM TREATMENT TO RECOVERY

In 1996, the U.S. Department of Health and Human Services (HHS) Center for Substance Abuse Treatment (CSAT) held its First National

Summit on Recovery. Over 100 invited stakeholders engaged in a variety of structured discussions to formulate a "recovery-oriented system of care" (CSAT, 2006, p. 6). The forum developed a definition of recovery: "Recovery from alcohol and drug problems is a process of change through which an individual achieves abstinence and improved health, wellness and quality of life" (CSAT, 2006, p. 9).

Twelve guiding principles of recovery were delineated. Most importantly, relapse was included as part of the process of recovery: "Recovery is not a linear process. It is based on continual growth and improved functioning. It may involve relapse and other setbacks, which are a natural part of the continuum but not inevitable outcomes. Wellness is the result of improved care and balance of mind, body and spirit. It is a product of the recovery process" (CSAT, 2006, p. 10–11). This represented a significant step forward in integrating the chronic and relapse-prone etiological formulation of addiction.

However, in my view, the summit's report presented an unfortunate omission. Strikingly absent was any reference to human sexuality, sexual health, or sexual behavior. Even though the 12 guiding principles of recovery include references to health and wellness—such as "the holistic nature of physical, mental, social, and spiritual changes experienced by an individual throughout recovery" (CSAT, 2006, p. 51)—it is noteworthy that sex is not overtly referenced anywhere in the 12 principles.

I believe that this omission reflects a broader lack within the current discussion of treatment and recovery. While great strides have been made in treating women and men suffering from addiction, their sexuality—particularly as a part of the recovery process—is marginalized and even made invisible. When sexuality is not directly and positively addressed in drug and alcohol treatment, it can contribute to treatment failure, relapse, and untold costs in the lives of addicts and their families.

Sexual Health in Drug and Alcohol Treatment is an evidence-based curriculum to provide lifelong sexual health–based recovery tools as part of the treatment experience.

FROM RECOVERY TO SEXUAL HEALTH IN RECOVERY

In 2001, I was at a party with my good friend and colleague Cheryl Houk, then executive director of Stepping Stone of San Diego, a residential drug and alcohol treatment center. "Too many of our residents are relapsing because of their sexual behavior," Cheryl declared. "We can do better." She wanted to find a way to address sexual behavior during and after treatment to "stop the dying" (C. Houk, personal communication, October 7, 2001).

I am a licensed marriage and family therapist specializing in treating men with out-of-control sexual behavior (OCSB) in San Diego for over 15 years. Over the years, several residents of Stepping Stone had been clients in my group and individual treatment program. These men were concurrently treating OCSB and their addiction. Cheryl knew of my work with the residents and wanted to discuss another problem at her center: crystal methamphetamine addiction. An increasing number of clients were presenting with crystal meth as their primary addiction. Over 75% of Stepping Stone clients identify as gay, lesbian, or bisexual, and crystal meth use is closely linked with sexual activity among gay males.

In Cheryl's view, the men with crystal meth addiction were bringing their sexual lives with them into treatment, and far too many were being forced to leave treatment as a result of violating program rules about sexual behavior. I remember asking Cheryl, "I wonder how often they stop giving people chemotherapy because of their sexual behavior at the hospital?"

Cheryl wanted my help. I offered to volunteer a few hours a month to assess the situation and offer recommendations. Our goal was to see why, after 6–9 months of living clean and sober, residents completed treatment only to relapse because of sexually motivated drug-using situations. Sometimes this relapse occurred within days or weeks of completing treatment. On a few tragic occasions, recently discharged residents were found dead of overdose.

It did not take us long to find there was indeed a significant subset of Stepping Stone residents whose treatment failure was inextricably linked with their sexual behavior. The residents included not only gay men who used meth but also women and men of all sexual orientations who combined all sorts of drugs and alcohol with sex. We quickly came to call this sex/drug-linked behavior. For many addicts, drug use prolonged their sexual activity and enhanced their libido. Others were able to pursue unconventional sexual habits only after using drugs. In recovery, residents missed these sexual activities, and their treatment program did not prepare them for the absence of this sexual intensity.

We discovered that a high percentage of sex/drug-linked residents failed to complete treatment. However, treatment failure was not always due to a drug relapse. Many times it was due to sexual behavior that violated treatment program policies.

Two coexisting problems began to emerge. First, the program lacked specific interventions for the increasing population of high sex/drug-linked addicts and alcoholics in treatment. Second, we realized that Stepping Stone relied on impulsive, judgmental, reactive, and outdated procedures in addressing sexual concerns among their residents.

For example, early in my consultation with Stepping Stone, a counselor requested my advice on how to respond to a sexual situation. A resident had found a roommate's sex toy that the roommate used for masturbation and had reported this to the counselor. For years, the policy at Stepping Stone was to confiscate sexual aids—and follow up with the resident in a (often humiliating) discussion about how such materials were not allowed at the residence.

I asked the staff to consider the ramifications of this policy. Clients of Stepping Stone live in the center for 6–9 months. "Is the expectation that Stepping Stone is an orgasm free zone?" I noted that clients were not given any positive sexual health messages about masturbation; it was only addressed when a boundary crossing, such as the possession of a sexual aid, occurred. (It was later discovered that the person who raised the issue was angry with the roommate and knew from experience that the staff would react swiftly and negatively; thus, the program's negative attitudes toward sexuality were used as a weapon of passive-aggressive retaliation among residents.)

In my opinion, this inability to address sexual concerns and issues does a disservice to both providers and clients. Some treatment providers are frustrated by the knowledge that their clients might have a better chance for recovery if sex/drug-linked behaviors are addressed more directly and thoroughly in treatment. Clients, who have assimilated recovery information and are ready to apply it to their lives, unfortunately remain at risk and often relapse because their treatment provided inadequate skills for navigating sexuality in recovery.

In my experience, Stepping Stone is not the only treatment program to mishandle sexual issues. Some drug and alcohol treatment centers operate under significantly outdated, ineffective, and disapproving views about sex. Sexuality is often addressed only when a client's sexual behavior conflicts with treatment program policies (e.g., those concerning HIV infection, sex between clients, sexual activity off grounds, falling in love with other clients).

Most drug and alcohol treatment programs do not have designated locations, groups, or interventions that provide clients with positive, affirming, and factual sexual health information. It is a rare chemical dependency treatment program that provides specialized programming for each client to explore, discuss, and understand how sexual behavior may possibly jeopardize recovery. Treatment fails these clients when they are not provided a safe place to discuss sexual health.

Furthermore, sexual health training is virtually absent in drug and alcohol treatment programs and counselor education training programs. The professional training of drug counselors focuses primarily on current treatment standards. Sex is only discussed in the context of HIV infection risk, pregnancy, history of sexual abuse, or possible co-occurring sex addiction (which is not the focus of this book). Many drug treatment professionals are directed by their supervisors and traditional treatment norms to limit any discussion of sexual concerns to these areas. If a client attempts to raise other sexual issues, it is a common drug treatment norm to classify such discussion as a deflection from treatment or something that the counselor is not competent to address.

Traditionally, alcohol and drug recovery centers have relegated addressing sexual behavior in early recovery to the back burner—or have believed that to address sexuality too soon in recovery risks client relapse. Chemical dependency treatment professionals often discuss sexual concerns from a sex negative or disease or pathology context. Therefore a client's sexual and relationship life is often limited to a focus on co-occurring sex addiction, sexually transmitted diseases, pregnancy, and/or the moral dimensions of conforming to an arbitrary set of sexual values and behaviors of specific staff or treatment programs. Additionally, the topic of sex is often taboo in the alcohol and drug treatment environment. Members of the staff have a difficult time broaching the subject. Chemical dependency treatment is inadequate and at times negligent when a client's sexual behavior, which is clearly linked with addictive drug use, is not carefully and thoroughly addressed in all phases of alcohol and drug treatment.

Cheryl Houk, her colleagues at Stepping Stone, and I began to realize that it did not matter how many treatment experiences high sex/drug-linked addicts had if their primary risk for relapse went untreated. At that time, Stepping Stone was no different than most treatment centers. Sex/drug-linked interventions were limited to a general recovery cultural norm of avoiding new relationships until a year sober. The slogan "sex took me out" was frequently mentioned by clients and provided us with an important lesson: the primary relapse prevention intervention was to make addicts become wary of sex and sexual desire. What seemed to be missing was a sexual health–based relapse prevention strategy. Could sexual health be inextricably linked with staying sober? A new treatment plan was needed.

SEXUAL HEALTH IN DRUG AND ALCOHOL TREATMENT: THE CURRICULUM

Sexual Health in Drug and Alcohol Treatment is a pioneering psycho-educational class providing a sexual health–based curriculum to reduce risk of relapse and increase client retention for men and women with sex/drug-linked addiction and alcoholism. It was created through a collaboration between drug and alcohol counselors, sexual health advocates, psychological/sexological research specialists, and more than 250 Stepping Stone clients who participated in the program. It is the first curriculum designed to integrate concepts of sexual health, current sex research, and recent developments in relapse prevention research.

I was honored to have Eli Coleman, PhD, professor and director of the Program in Human Sexuality, Department of Family Practice and Community Health, at the University of Minnesota Medical School, Chris Kraft, PhD, Johns Hopkins Center for Marital and Sexual Health, Sexual Behaviors Consultation Unit, and Stephanie Covington, PhD, LCSW, codirector of the Institute for Relational Development in La Jolla, California serve as an external review committee. They gave me feedback, reactions, and suggestions as well as critique. They were instrumental in the developmental trajectory of the curriculum in its current form.

The curriculum is not a specialty program for clients with sexual problems. The curriculum is designed for *all* drug and alcohol treatment acuity levels. For it to be effective, each and every client in the treatment program must attend the class.

The curriculum originated in 2003, when the California Endowment funded a 3-year grant for Stepping Stone to develop, implement, and measure treatment outcomes of a sexual health–based, harm-reduction, relapse-prevention program targeted at sex/drug-linked addiction. The goal was to improve client retention rates and decrease sex/drug-linked relapse during all phases of treatment. I wrote the initial curriculum as the structure for the weekly psychoeducational sexual health in recovery group.

Theoretical Basis of the Curriculum

This curriculum is founded in three complementary theories, the most central being the transtheoretical model of change and motivational enhancement approaches that facilitate the change process (Miller & Rollnick, 1991; Prochaska, Norcross, & DiClemente, 1994). The readiness for change process is an excellent match for the necessary suspension of judgment and client-centered approach that is central to initial client engagement in addressing sexual health concerns among substance abusers (Braun-Harvey, 1997). The curriculum integrates a variety of change processes that are fundamental to the theoretical structure of the stages of readiness for change model (Prochaska et al., 1994).

Second, sexual health in recovery is a harm-reduction technique for improving abstinence-based recovery. Harm-reduction strategies are often utilized in nonabstinence-based substance abusing treatment approaches or to address substance abuse problems among precontemplators (Denning, 2000). Harm-reduction approaches are integrated within the curriculum by approaching sexual health as harm reduction. Building sexual health skills within the recovery process will reduce the risk of relapse. However, sexual health in recovery is not an all-or-nothing behavior (like complete abstinence from drugs and/or alcohol). Sexual health is a process of change incorporating sexual health behaviors, attitudes, and understanding that support the recovery process.

Last, the curriculum utilizes cognitive-behavioral learning principles that have been applied to other conditions, such as depression and anxiety management. Affect regulation skills are an important component of mental health. Thoughts and feelings in response to sexual situations are significant relapse risks at many stages of recovery. The curriculum is designed to be applicable to men and women at various stages of the recovery process. It is not limited to initial treatment or acute treatment settings. The cognitive-behavioral skill sets for each of the 12 curriculum lessons are designed for repeated practice. Sexual health is a process of change, not an event. The curriculum reflects this basic principle of recovery.

The structure of the psychoeducational group provides the container in which participants can experience feelings about their individual sexuality. Sessions are designed to raise consciousness about sexual health; each class is an exercise in sexual self-reevaluation. Each session provides an opportunity for clients to understand more about their sexual selves.

The most important task in this reevaluation process is to continually connect recovery with sexual health. Sexuality as an ally in recovery, rather than an adversary, is a central treatment frame. The curriculum helps women and men in recovery to identify sexual thoughts and feelings associated with increasing or decreasing risk of relapse. Several of the sessions emphasize the importance of not prematurely entering sexual situations without adequate preparation and consideration of recovery. The repetitive nature of the skill-building exercises allow for an ongoing commitment to sexual health in recovery that will be evidenced by repeat usage of the recovery tools over months and years of recovery.

Most sexual health discussions will arouse a wide variety of emotions within each participant as well as within the group; these emotions are an important part of the change process. A central element of the curriculum is to present a sex-positive attitude about sex and recovery. Sexual health in recovery is being deeply committed to believing in one's ability to maintain recovery and have an active, pleasurable, and emotionally meaningful sexual life. Of primary importance is reducing shame associated with choosing to avoid a sexual situation or emotional circumstance that will elevate risk of relapse to an unmanageable level. It is only through sex-positive, shame-reduction interactions that men and women in recovery will increasingly seek out relationships that support the goals of abstinence and sexual health.

Implementation of the Curriculum

The pioneering nature of this intervention required the development of two new drug and alcohol treatment tools. Dr. Jim Zians developed for Stepping Stone an assessment survey for determining each client's level of relapse risk linked to sexual behavior; this survey was also used to develop an evidence-based outcome evaluation process. The assessment survey was given to each resident upon admission and thereafter at 3-month intervals. The survey determined each resident's level of sex/drug relapse risk by evaluating factors such as: client drug use, sex/drug-linked behavior, influences of cognitive and interpersonal style, frequency and intensity of sexual secrets and shame, pervasiveness of negative sexual health attitudes, and frequency of risky sexual practices. Clients were given feedback by the sexual behavior relapse prevention specialist, a professional who was trained to conduct the assessment and feedback session.

From November 2003 to May 2007, more than 250 Stepping Stone residents completed the initial assessment survey. Residents completed a second survey following 3 months of residential treatment, during which they attended weekly sexual health in recovery group sessions. The group sessions were attended by every Stepping Stone client during that period; group attendance was not based on client level of sex/drug-linked relapse risk. Attendance was a required component of the program. Additional program components included one-on-one counseling sessions for residents assessed to be a high relapse risk because of sex/drug-linked addiction patterns.

Concurrently, numerous staff trainings, programmatic changes, and ongoing staff supervision of sexual health interventions, policy, and group sessions were held to develop sex-positive treatment norms and to ensure that the curriculum content was integrated within the entire treatment program. Eventually, the sexual health in recovery group sessions were provided free to Stepping Stone outpatient clients and the greater San Diego recovery community. Several other mental health programs in San Diego have now incorporated the initial Stepping Stone curriculum within their overall clinical services. Meanwhile, Stepping Stone has become the go-to treatment center in San Diego for addressing crystal meth and other drugs and their link with sexual behavior. The curriculum is so integrated within their programming that even though almost every staff member involved in the 2002 pilot program has moved on, the commitment to sexual health based recovery remains unwavering.

Format of the Curriculum

The curriculum in this book differs in several ways from the 2003 original. I have added components based on client and staff feedback as well as the latest sexual health research. However, the original structure (four core themes, each taught in three focused lessons) remains.

This version includes more experiential learning than the initial version, which relied too heavily on cognitive learning and group process. It lacked sufficient variety of psychoeducational group formats to meet the diverse learning styles of men and women in treatment. Thus, each of the 12 sessions begins with a brief lecture followed by an expanded experiential learning group process. This is the heart of each session. Experiential learning allows for a group process to unfold within a structured task completion, either as the full group or as separate gender or relationship status groups. The final lesson section, "Topic Skill Practice," creates an opportunity for each group to work with a sexual health skill set and practice completing a recovery tool worksheet. This is another shame-reduction intervention. Feeling ignorant, uninformed, or awkward about sexual information is an enormous barrier to sexual health discussions. The practice session provides a shared moment of vulnerability and openness. This group process is done in the context of learning how to fill out the sheet while serving a central function for improving treatment outcomes for high sex/drug-linked participants: reducing sex/drug linked shame.

Implementing the Curriculum at Stepping Stone

As mentioned earlier, *Sexual Health in Drug and Alcohol Treatment* was tested at Stepping Stone. Founded in 1976, Stepping Stone currently operates both a residential and a nonresidential nonprofit social model recovery program in San Diego, California. The residential program is located in an urban residential neighborhood in central San Diego. Stepping Stone relies on the 12 steps of Alcoholics Anonymous and peer interaction and involvement to create a social environment where clients help each other in the recovery process. Stepping Stone has a reputation for integrating new approaches to treatment.

The residential program provides treatment for 28 adults, 75% of whom identify as lesbian, gay, bisexual or transgender and who voluntarily self-identify with drug or alcohol dependency. More than half of the men in treatment are living with HIV infection.

During the program evaluation period (2003–2007), the client demographics of the sexual health in recovery program reflected the general demographics of San Diego. Clients were White (60%), Latino/a (16%), and African American (7%), with the rest being Asian-Pacific Islander, Native American, or biracial. More than 70% of the study participants were between 25 and 44 years old.

Stepping Stone relies on a large volunteer program to provide daily support for residents. The staff is composed primarily of paraprofessionals and certified drug and alcoholism counselors; most have high school diploma or bachelor degree. Three master's-level counselors who had just completed their schooling taught the curriculum to the sexual health in recovery group. I supervised the implementation of the curriculum and trained the staff, but they did the work. None of the staff had specialized training in human sexuality; in fact, only one of the three group facilitators had taken any advanced sexuality coursework at a master's degree level.

One of the most encouraging and inspiring outcomes of this project was seeing the Stepping Stone counselors, staff, volunteers, and administration enthusiastically integrate the curriculum and recommended program changes. The sexual health in recovery project was presented as a pioneering opportunity to see if changing from a sex-negative to a sex-positive treatment environment could improve client recovery and retention; it also met head-on the pervasive feeling of hopelessness that had permeated the program surrounding crystal meth and other sex/drug-linked addictions.

The experience at Stepping Stone has increased my belief that sexual health is an aspiration for almost everyone in recovery. This curriculum can be taught by a wide variety of drug and alcohol professionals; the only requirement for leading the course are personal qualities of non-judgmental open-minded curiosity about sexual health in all its facets. The enthusiastic implementation of this curriculum at Stepping Stone significantly challenges the current orthodoxy that drug counselors cannot address issues of sexual health within recovery.

The wonderful staff at Stepping Stone demonstrated to me that there is a tremendous hunger for sexual health recovery tools among drug and alcoholism professionals. Their dedication to learning and changing was an inspiration. As for the clients, the residents of Stepping Stone embraced this program with excitement, relief, and increasing confidence in their ability to stay sober. They finally had a place to talk about sex and drugs! The men and women whose lives were on the edge of destruction before entering treatment were not to be underestimated. From the first day of the experiment they looked forward to the class and were so grateful to be in a treatment program where sexuality was positively addressed rather than feared and avoided.

Most importantly, Stepping Stone found sexual behavioral problems within the treatment center plummet after implementation of the program. We theorized that when you provide a place for sexual health discussions, it eliminates the need for sexual issues to spill out in other rooms or places.

In September 2008, a news program on the sexual health in recovery program at Stepping Stone included an interview with Gabriel, a 30-year-old gay male crystal meth addict who had just completed 6 months of the program. "I was learning to be in touch with Gabriel, with me, my body, how to communicate what my needs were, how to communicate what I wanted," he said in the interview. "[As a crystal meth addict] I had learned a whole way of living where all of my safer sex practices had gone out the window and my self-esteem had gone out the window. . . . I had to rebuild that from scratch" (Goldberg, 2008).

Evaluating the Curriculum

The sexual health in recovery curriculum was developed as part of a grant from the California Endowment. The grant funded a 3-year evolution of this program through conception, design, implementation, evaluation, and outcome data. Jim Zians, PhD, rigorously expected every component of the program to be measurable before we began. Thus the Stepping Stone curriculum was part of a well-designed, evidence-based program.

As mentioned earlier, Zians developed a client assessment survey for Stepping Stone, which not only gave us greater definition and clarity into the problem of sex/drug-linked relapse but also provided an excellent outcome measure to determine if the program met our goals: increased client retention and decreased client relapse due to sex/drug-linked behavior. The most important treatment outcome, in our opinion, was client retention. When men and women with high sex/drug-linked relapse risk complete treatment that includes a sexual health relapse prevention program they increase the likelihood of remaining abstinent and engaged in recovery.

The survey also included measures of psychological constructs related to positive outcomes for residential substance abuse treatment. Several measures were adapted to survey targeted behaviors and attitudes specific to treatment outcomes related to sex/drug-linked patterns of use. The survey also measured sexual health attitudes and behaviors, especially those connected with the client's anticipation of treatment completion given his or her history of sex/drug-linked behavior. Depression, anxiety, and other symptoms associated with mental disorders were included.

The most salient measure turned out to be an assessment of shame and stigma associated with sex/drug-linked history and current behavior: the Personal Feelings Questionnaire (PFQ) (Harder & Lewis, 1987), a validated measure of proneness to shame and guilt. I proposed to Dr. Zians that a measure for shame was essential for the overall survey, given the debilitating sexual shame I had witnessed in my work with men and out-of-control sexual behavior. Jim chose the PFQ for its flexibility and adaptability to create additional items that describe shame associated with sex/drug-linked behavior (e.g., "I often think about a sexual secret I hide from others"; "I worry that some aspect of my sexual behavior may cause me problems with my program at Stepping Stone"). The PFQ also asks about the frequency of subjective body sensations and emotional states of shame without naming or labeling the sensation as "shame" (e.g., "feeling ridiculous," "laughable," "humiliated," "stupid," and "childish").

Since Stepping Stone serves primarily lesbian, gay, bisexual, and transgender adults, an outness measure was included to distinguish shame between sex/drug-linked activity and that which might stem from sexual identity development and behavior of sexual orientation. It was filled out by self-identified lesbian, gay, bisexual, or transgender residents.

It was unclear how prevalent co-occurring symptoms of sexual risk taking, HIV infection risk, or HIV virus transmission risk and compulsive sexual behavior were among low or high sex/drug-linked addicts at Stepping Stone. Thus the assessment integrated components of sexual sensation–seeking measures, condom use, safer sex boundaries, as well as symptoms associated with out-of-control sexual behavior.

A modified measure based on readiness for change with a focus on the preparation and action stage of change was included to address motivation for change and self-efficacy. Since sexual health in recovery is based on the transtheoretical model (TTM) of change, we were interested in motivational readiness for addressing sexual health in drug and alcohol treatment (e.g., "When I feel my problem behavior coming on I think about it or go talk to someone at Stepping Stone about it, I feel more confident that my sexual behavior will not lead to relapse").

Dr. Zians and I coordinated the development of the curriculum and assessment in tandem. His mantra was, "If I can't measure it, it can't be in the curriculum." The curriculum was developed with specific constructs associated with recovery and sexual health. These constructs included sexual attitudes and beliefs, peer attitudes and beliefs, stage of readiness for change, skill efficacy (can I and do I believe I can implement sexual health in recovery skills and practices?), self regulation (how does sexual health in recovery contribute to the process of moving from a large scale breakdown in self-regulation to increasingly stronger levels of self-regulation?), and of course shame (how does a client's self-reported level of shame contribute to increasing or decreasing his or her risk of sex/drug relapse?).

Each time a resident completed a survey, the Stepping Stone staff completed a one-page evaluation using chart entries from the client's file.

Entries included such information as: changes in HIV status, a recently acquired sexually transmitted infection (STI), number of sexual health in recovery groups attended, number of individual counseling sessions with the sexual behavior relapse prevention specialist, and, most importantly, staff opinion ratings on program compliance and sex/drug-linked relapse risk during the measurement period. We were interested in the correlation between staff perceptions of sex/drug-linked relapse and the residents' own self-reports of relapse risk.

At 3 months and 6 months, each resident was given the same assessment with one addition: a confidential Behavior Outcome Questionnaire, which addressed drug use, sexual behavior, and sex/drug-linked behavior over the previous 3 months. The outcome data from this assessment hinged on Stepping Stone agreeing to a privacy boundary they had never before been asked to consider: would program staff be willing to allow Dr. Zians to anonymously know resident drug use over the past 3 months (from the questionnaire) and *not* require him to disclose that information? In other words, any anonymous self-reported relapse or sexual behavior by clients, as recounted on the questionnaire, would *not* be reported to the program staff. After much consideration, the staff at Stepping Stone agreed to this. Thus, the results from two measures—the Behavior Outcome Questionnaire and a client satisfaction measure—were kept confidential from program staff.

It should be noted that a different boundary was established regarding suicidal risk or acute psychiatric symptoms that might become evident in some of the psychological measures. The sexual behavior relapse prevention counselor checked one question pertaining to suicidality prior to implementing the confidentiality procedures, thus assuring that clients deemed in need of care would come to the attention of the staff.

Evaluation Results

Two significant evaluation outcomes warrant attention. First, client retention improved by over 50% when compared with the 3 years prior to the implementation of the sexual health relapse prevention program. This is important given that a primary goal of the intervention was to stem the increasing number of premature discharges due to sex/drug-linked relapse. This suggests to us that sex/drug-linked behaviors are learned. By adopting a sexual health–based model of treatment combined with clinical interventions (psychoeducational curriculum, drug/sex-linked relapse prevention skill practice, and self-reflection experiences), these learned responses could be separated, and, over time, clients would have increased confidence in their ability to sustain sexual activity and relations without jeopardizing their recovery.

Second, assessment measures revealed a strikingly salient risk factor: sex/drug-linked shame. Stepping Stone residents assessed to be at highest risk for sex/drug-linked relapse entered treatment with *double* the measured levels of shame when compared with the lower risk sex/drug-linked clients. Three months later, after completing the first of two cycles of the Stepping Stone curriculum, this high-risk group lowered their shame levels to the same range as clients who entered treatment with low sex/drug-linked histories. Thus, *Sexual Health in Drug and Alcohol Treatment* is a shame-reduction intervention that provides sexual health–based relapse prevention tools.

A commitment to integrating sexual health into drug and alcohol treatment is a comprehensive endeavor. This text will outline the client intervention. The forthcoming book *Sexual Health in Recovery* (Springer Publishing Company) will address the process of integrating sex/drug-linked, sexual health-based relapse prevention into all aspects of treatment and recovery.

REACTIONS TO SEXUAL HEALTH IN RECOVERY

I have presented trainings and workshops on the sexual health in recovery program since 2003, in forums as diverse as: the Society for the Scientific Study of Sexuality (SSSS); the American Association of Sexuality Educators, Counselors and Therapists (AASECT); the Society for the Advancement of Sexual Health (SASH); the National Conference on Methamphetamine, HIV and Hepatitis; Hazelden Graduate School; the California Association of Marriage and Family Therapists (CAMFT); the California Association of Drug and Alcohol Counselors (CAADAC); the National Association of Addiction Treatment Providers (NAATP); the American Psychiatric Association (APA); the Maryland State Office of AIDS; and the Whitman Walker Clinic in Washington, DC. At nearly every presentation, attendees endorse the curriculum and its challenging of entrenched traditional drug treatment sexual behavior messages. The most common question I get is, "When will the curriculum be available?"

In 2008, I co-presented a session at the Western Regional SSSS with David B. Wohlsifer, PhD, a Pennsylvania sex researcher. Dr. Wohlsifer conducted qualitative interviews and analyzed the sexual beliefs and behaviors of six men who have had sex with other men while using crystal methamphetamine (CMSM) for his doctoral dissertation. Although entirely unrelated to our research (at the time, Dr. Wohlsifer was unaware of this curriculum), his findings supported our outcome findings: "Shame about their homosexual sexual behavior appeared to play a key role in motivating these men to use crystal. Crystal seemed to provide an escape from sexual shame. Sex Positive Cognitive Therapy is suggested as an optimal treatment model for CMSM" (Wohlsifer, 2006, p. iv). Dr. Wohlsifer concluded that

> treatment research needs to be sex positive especially in areas related to crystal use. What I have learned from these six men is that crystal either facilitated or mitigated their sexual encounters. They were able to be sexual, and enjoy sex with other men, which made using the drug all the more appealing. The crystal induced alternate state of sexual reality was far more enticing than its sober shame based alternative. Thus to respond to the community health problems that crystal use presents, it is essential to understand that crystal use is a mechanism that eradicates sexual shame. (Wohlsifer, 2006, p. 53)

IMPLEMENTING SEXUAL HEALTH IN RECOVERY AT YOUR FACILITY

The positive outcomes of the sexual health in drug and alcohol treatment at Stepping Stone suggest that this curriculum is a new resource for a subset of treatment-seeking clients whose sexual shame is an unseen treatment barrier. All levels of addiction treatment can implement this curriculum in an existing treatment program. It will, however, require a commitment to acquiring skills in sexual health–based treatment approaches as well as addressing program policies and entrenched patterns of ignoring or denying sex/drug-linked relapse risks.

Compatibility With Existing Treatment Programs

Although it was developed within a residential and outpatient social model 12-step treatment program, sexual health in drug and alcohol treatment is not based on the 12 steps of Alcoholics Anonymous. It is a harm-reduction, cognitive-learning, sexual health–based intervention that can be conducted in a wide variety of treatment programs.

The curriculum is founded on an abstinence-based treatment model where sex/drug-linked behavior is addressed to mitigate relapse from an abstinence-based approach to recovery.

Program Clientele

The program does not espouse sexual values founded on any particular religious creed or belief; it is based on sexual science and concepts of sexual health. Thus, men and women from any religious background, from devout believer to atheist, can participate in sexual health in drug and alcohol treatment groups.

The program was developed in a treatment environment in which heterosexual clients were the minority; the majority of Stepping Stone's clients were lesbian, gay, bisexual, or transgender men and women. This unique setting provided for daily evidence that this curriculum is not limited to a specific sexual orientation, gender, or socioeconomic circumstance. Stepping Stone treated homeless and unemployed clients, as well as well educated, wealthy clients who had lost everything in their addiction. Sexual health became another great equalizer among the treatment community.

Stepping Stone agreed with my recommendation to have the sexual health in recovery group be a required component of treatment for every resident and outpatient client. I think this was a fortuitous decision; I could well imagine the potential embarrassment of clients who were singled out to attend the special sex class. This split would create an anti-sexual health environment. The necessary message is that everyone in recovery needs to learn about sexual health; those with high sex/drug-linked patterns merely have more at stake.

Program Schedule

The curriculum is composed of an orientation, plus weekly lessons, each of which takes 90 minutes to implement; thus the entire program can be taught in a minimum of 13 weeks. Each lesson is self-contained; skills and topics do appear in more than one lesson but are not prerequisites for future lessons. This allows for creativity in adapting topics, schedules, and targeted sexual health skills within a wide variety of treatment settings. The curriculum can be one component of a comprehensive treatment program; it can also be offered as a separate treatment service, with enormous potential for community outreach and education. (For example, Stepping Stone continues to offer community-based groups for men and women who long ago completed an inpatient or outpatient treatment program.)

Staff Requirements and Preparation

This curriculum can be led by a skilled psychoeducational group leader with basic sexuality education and an interest in learning about sexual health. As mentioned earlier, at Stepping Stone the class was taught by master's-level counselors who were just embarking on their professional careers. None of the staff had specialized training in human sexuality; in fact, only one of the three group facilitators had taken any sexuality coursework at a master's degree level. A high level of comfort and openness when discussing sexuality and sexual topics is essential to convey the sex-positive message of the curriculum.

Stepping Stone spent a year preparing to implement this program. They conducted surveys to find out what the residents would find valuable in such a program. In addition, top leadership staff attended monthly sexual health meetings that I facilitated to discuss their own ambivalent feelings and attitudes about embarking on this venture. Consensus was difficult, and fears needed to be respected and addressed.

They did not have any path to guide their way. There was no one to pick up the phone and ask, How did you decide to write your statement of affirming sexuality? What is your approach to providing masturbation guidelines for gay men sharing rooms with heterosexual men? What programmatic sexual health responses do you implement when two residents form an attraction?

How long would it take to implement this program in your treatment setting? It depends on your goals. The most significant variable I can suggest is how well-entrenched sex-negative attitudes and policies are within your current treatment program. The more frequently you feel discouraged by current approaches to sexuality in treatment, or the more often discussions of sexuality are met with age-old defenses common among drug treatment professionals, the more time you may want to take in implementing the curriculum.

Stepping Stone learned this lesson in a surprisingly harsh manner. A female Stepping Stone resident needed to transfer to another local treatment center. She had attended numerous sexual health in recovery groups and had enjoyed the general open and honest sexual discussions related to recovery that were daily occurrences there. In her interview with the program director at the new treatment program, she took out her skill set sheets from the sexual health in recovery group and asked who in the program would support her in continuing this work. The director clenched her fist, pounded it on the desk, and said, "We don't talk about sex here!"

SUMMARY

As the sexual health in recovery program proceeded at Stepping Stone, a general tone of sexual knowledge and information permeated attitudes and discussions not only with clients but also among staff. The volunteers, paraprofessionals, drug counselors, and professional staff took pride in their developing competence and confidence in engaging in matters of sexual health. However, it was not an easy or one-way trajectory. I have enormous respect for the difficult conversations, risks, conflicts, and disagreements that took place as we moved toward sex-positive treatment.

One of our most surprising findings was that the staff (many of whom were also in recovery) began to envy the residents. They remembered their own struggles with sexual health in recovery and saw how this issue had been neglected in their own treatment. This created many poignant moments of tears and healing. I was privileged to earn their trust and confidence as a consultant and facilitator for implementing the program as well as supporting their own recovery process.

Stepping Stone had to navigate the antisexual attitudes common to a wide variety of treatment programs. Their resolve never waned. They continue to be the biggest advocate of sexual health–based recovery in the country, and for that they are to be applauded. However, their hard work will be for naught if you, having read this far, decide "well, it's not for me." Had this been the response of Cheryl Houk, I would not have written this curriculum. More importantly, there would not be several dozen men and women grateful to be alive.

On my last consultation, after 3 years of groundbreaking work, I overheard a conversation between a recently hired female counselor and a female resident. The worried resident initiated the conversation. She had been masturbating in her room the previous day and had an arousing fantasy involving her former drug using partner. She was concerned about this and had learned in the sex class not to keep these worries to herself. The staff member was poised, welcoming, and first and foremost congratulated the resident for caring enough about her sobriety to proactively address a sex/drug-linked relapse risk. I am convinced that such a conversation would not have been possible prior to implementing the curriculum at Stepping Stone, and that conversations such as this can make the difference in helping a client achieve and maintain sobriety. I hope that this curriculum helps other treatment programs achieve the same level of awareness, openness and comfort in discussing sexual issues and their relation to recovery.

REFERENCES

Braun-Harvey, D. (1997). Sexual dependence among recovering substance-abusing men. In S. L. A. Straussner & E. Zelvin (Eds.), *Gender and addictions: Men and women in treatment* (pp. 359–384). Northvale, NJ: Jason Aronson Inc.
Center for Substance Abuse Treatment (CSAT). (2006). *National Summit on Recovery: Conference report* (DHHS Publication No. [SMA] 06-xxxx). Rockville, MD: Substance Abuse and Mental Health Services Administration.
Childress, A., Mozley, D., McElgin, W., Fitzgerald, J., Reivich, M., & O'Brien, C. (1999). Limbic activation during cue-induced cocaine craving. *American Journal of Psychiatry, 156,* 11–18.
Denning, P. (2000). *Practicing harm reduction psychotherapy: An alternative approach to addictions.* New York: The Guilford Press.
Goldberg, K. (2008). *Local program uses instruction on sexual health to help people recover from drug addiction.* Retrieved March 12, 2008, from http://www.kpbs.org/news/local;id=12670.
Gordon, S. (2003). *Relapse & recovery: Behavioral strategies for change.* Wernersville, PA: Caron Treatment Centers.
Harder, D. W., & Lewis, S. J. (1987). Additional construct validity evidence for the Harder Personal Feelings Questionnaire measure of shame and guilt proneness. *Psychological Reports, 67,* 288–290.
Lesher, (2003). Science is revolutionizing our view of addiction—and what to do about it *Focus, 1,* 194–195.
Marcelle, G. (2006). *Drug scope: Drug data update focus: Myths about methamphetamine November 30, 2006.* Retrieved February 7, 2009, from http://drugscope.blogspot.com/2006/11/focus-us-myths-about-methamphetamine_30.html
McLellan, T. (2007). *Treatment is over. Now what if a relapse happens?* Retrieved March 12, 2009, from http://www.hbo.com/addiction/aftercare/48_what_if_a_relapse_hap pens.html
Miller, W. R., & Rollnick, S. (1991). *Motivational interviewing: Preparing people to change addictive behavior.* New York: The Guilford Press.
National Institute on Alcohol Abuse and Alcoholism (NIAAA). (1996). *NIAAA reports Project MATCH main findings.* Retrieved February 6, 2009, from http://www.niaaa.nih.gov/NewsEvents/NewsReleases/match.htm
Prochaska, J. O., Norcross, J. C., & DiClemente, C. C. (1994). *Changing for good.* New York: Avon Books.

Project MATCH Research Group. (1993). Project MATCH: Rationale and methods for a multisite clinical trial matching patients to alcoholism treatment. *Alcoholism: Clinical and Experimental Research, 17*, 1130–1145.

Volkow, N. D., Fowler, J. S., Wolf, A. P., Schlyer, D., Shiue, C. Y., Alpert, R., et al. (1999). Association of methylphenidate-induced craving with changes in right striato-orbit-ofrontal metabolism in cocaine abusers: Implications in addiction. *American Journal of Psychiatry, 156*, 19–26.

Wohlsifer, D. B. (2006). *An examination of the sexological aspects of men who have sex with men and use crystal methamphetamine.* Unpublished doctoral dissertation, the Institute for Advanced Study of Human Sexuality, San Francisco, California.

Note to Group Leader

A vital component for quality group work is leader preparation. Long before clients gather for their first group, the well-prepared leader will have spent hours readying not only for the first session but also for the many meetings yet to come. Most problems in new groups stem from inadequate leader preparation.

The suggestions and observations I put forth here come from 25 years as a group therapist, workshop leader, trainer, consultant, and classroom instructor—as well as the 4 years I worked on the design and implementation of the sexual health in recovery program at Stepping Stone in San Diego. I hope you find these suggestions useful and informative. In providing them, I have tried to answer the question: What is essential to start the group, and what is necessary to be adequately prepared?

MISSION STATEMENT

Why Do You Want to Lead This Group?

This is the first question that must be answered by every person preparing to facilitate this unique program. Sexual health in drug and alcohol treatment is a cutting edge curriculum; the group leaders who facilitate the sessions will be the primary voice and face for sexual health in recovery at the treatment center. Why were you selected? Why did you agree? It is important to formulate a statement that represents your motivation, interest, and commitment to learning this program and adapting it for your specific treatment setting and population. Your mission statement will support you during both the exhilarating days and the exhausting days of leading this group.

As discussed in the introduction, sexuality and recovery have been wary housemates for a long time. As the group leader, you will be the primary mediator for these two distrustful factions. Sexual health in recovery is a tool to structure this much-needed dialogue. I hope this curriculum inspires you to become a voice within drug and alcohol treatment to reduce relapse by bridging sexual health with recovery.

PROGRAM GOALS

In 2002, when we set out to create this intervention, we were supported by a grant from the California Endowment. From the very beginning, the staff at Stepping Stone, myself, and the program evaluator agreed on our key goals for the program. These were crucial in order to ultimately determine whether we were successful.

You may not be conducting a funded program, but I do think a clear statement from the leadership of your treatment program—one which outlines what you hope to accomplish, especially in the first year or two—is necessary. In our case, Stepping Stone wanted to improve client retention by 50% over 3 years and decrease treatment termination following sexually linked drug use.

What are your program goals? Are they realistic? Is there general agreement among the leadership of your organization? This will be very important when the program comes under scrutiny. And it will. Sexual health challenges the status quo, and change is difficult. People become ambivalent when they feel they are being required change too much. When treatment involves integration of sexuality, the discomfort of professional staff, counselors, program leaders, and clients can at times be quite palpable. However, if your organization has established goals for the program, the unforeseen challenges and difficulties will be girded by these overall goals. Bumps in the road are an indication of change—not that something is inherently wrong. Hold on to your mission. Remain steadfast in sexual health as an ally in drug and alcohol treatment.

PREPARATION FOR THE PROGRAM

As a group therapist and one who trains group therapists, I have become convinced that preparation is vital to the success of the early life of group. First, read the entire curriculum. Second, read the required readings for all 12 lessons. Then, meet with key members of your treatment center and discuss what you liked best about the curriculum and what you have reservations about. Struggling alone with your doubts is sure to misfire. Trusted leaders and supervisors at your treatment center need to understand your excitement—and your caution. This will keep the rose-colored glasses well out of reach. These dialogues will keep your enthusiasm grounded in reality. Address major concerns before proceeding.

At Stepping Stone, we had to address unexpected envy among the staff and volunteers who were formerly program residents who had been in treatment many years ago. They were envious that the current clients were getting something they had not. Some of them had suffered greatly because a program like sexual health in drug and alcohol treatment did not exist when they were in treatment. Listening to their pain as they remembered (for some) hidden stories about their own sex/drug-linked behavior and having no place to discuss this was humbling and strengthened everyone's resolve to do this professionally, passionately, and respectfully. Basically, after these conversations it was clear that no one wanted to see the program fail.

PROGRAM LOGISTICS

Central to the initial success of this program is attention to detail. For example, when Stepping Stone had the group participants sit in rows instead of a circle, classroom management concerns became almost nonexistent. When we started sexual health in drug and alcohol treatment we did not know yet what a central role shame and shame reduction would play in reducing sex/drug-linked relapse. It was only after the evaluation measures demonstrated the importance of shame that we figured out why sitting in a circle was associated with so much disruptive client behavior.

Shame is first felt in expressions of others; we see our own shame in other people's faces. It was asking too much of the participants to learn important relapse prevention skills, discuss sexuality, discuss sex/drug-linked relapse, process the feeling they were experiencing in a psychoeducational group format, and to have them deal with the facial expressions of more than 25 other group members! So after some brainstorming between myself, the group leaders, and the program director, we arranged the chairs in rows, like a classroom. (We only employed circles when we conducted smaller, separate men's and women's groups in certain lessons.) This worked wonderfully.

So be flexible; let yourself adapt as you learn what works and what may need evaluation.

It also helps to set expectations for all participants. Your program probably has well-established cultural and treatment norms for your groups. However, sexual health in drug and alcohol treatment will raise discussions of sex and sexuality not only in group sessions but also, probably, throughout the remainder of your treatment program. This is normal; ideally sexuality should be integrated within the fabric of treatment. So how do you handle client discussions and possible privacy issues? For example, at Stepping Stone a client wanted to discuss his success with managing a boundary about masturbation with his roommate by talking about it in group. (In that particular case, the roommates agreed on a boundary of not discussing masturbation issues with other clients to embarrass each other.) Where will these conversations take place? What staff will listen and see the value of addressing a boundary challenge as a recovery tool?

So, in the first year, no detail is too small. Think critically. Think clearly. Ask questions. Plan. Write it down. By attending to the details, you will be able to release your creativity in leading the group sessions.

THE CURRICULUM

This is not a traditional curriculum; it is formatted as an actual script. Traditionally a curriculum is a structured guide of the psychoeducational process and does not provide so much of what is actually spoken. My experience with writing the curriculum led me to this choice.

DO I NEED TO FOLLOW THE SCRIPT?

The first time you teach each of the 12 sessions, I suggest following the script as closely as possible. You have enough to attend to without having to know all your lines. I think it also serves to reassure the clients. They know you are new at this. They know it is a new program. After all, most treatment centers probably do not offer this service (at least not for quite a while!). When clients observe you using the words of the invisible sex expert, it will add a sense of professionalism. They know someone who must know a lot about this is in the room as well, even though they will never meet. This was my boundary as a consultant at Stepping Stone. I did not teach the class. I trained facilitators to teach the sessions.

Find a mentor who can observe a few sessions (not the first five or six sessions, however, or the clients will think the observer is there to watch them) and ask for facilitative feedback. As your group facilitation becomes more confident, you can begin to develop your own style in working with the content.

I hope the script provides solid footing, and that over time, you are able to integrate your sexual health language within the individual learning elements for each lesson. The fundamentals, however, must remain. They are:

- The core concept
- Belief statement
- Objectives
- Change goals
- Opening sequence (which is repeated in each lesson)
- Clear delineation between lecture, experiential learning, and topic skill practice
- Closing

These elements must always remain as the core structure. It is this reliable structure and framework that will allow the sexual health group to be sustained week after week. An adequate container must be established and maintained so the group can become a working group. (Lesson 11, "Sexual Boundaries in Recovery," is a good reminder of these basics for safety and health.)

Components of the Curriculum

Here is a brief explanation of each section of the lesson:

- The "Core Concept" explains the key point of the lesson.
- The "Belief Statement" explains the link between the sexual health lesson and its implications for recovery.
- "Objectives" are the goals that each participant should achieve during the lesson.
- "Change Goals" are changes in participant's attitudes, knowledge, or beliefs that will result from participating in the lesson.

- "Required Reading for Group Leader" is background material on which the lesson is based. This will provide you with important background on the underlying theories and research behind each lesson and will also give you greater confidence to address the material with the group.
- "Recommended Materials for Group Leader" are additional books, articles, Web sites, and multimedia offerings that, while not essential, will help increase your understanding of the material and the concerns of men and women in recovery.
- "Required Materials for the Lesson" is a list of items you will need to have on hand prior to each lesson. In many cases these include copies of worksheets and/or handouts that are included at the end of every lesson.
- The "Opening" allows participants to settle themselves and prepare for the lesson. It includes music, an opening statement from the group leader, and a brief poem or reading.
- The "Group Introduction" is identical in every lesson. It reminds participants of the goals of the sexual health in recovery group.
- The "Lesson Introduction" introduces the main point and goal of each lesson.
- The "Lecture" is a brief discussion by the group leader. Throughout the lecture and following components, instructions to the group leader (not to be read aloud to the group) are indicated in *italic*.
- "Experiential Learning" includes exercises designed to help the group understand and experience the information presented in the lecture.
- "Topic Skill Practice" offers participants a chance to practice the skills they have learned in the lesson and practice completion of the recovery tool worksheet for each lesson.
- The "Closing" allows the leader a chance to refocus and center the participants before they leave the group.

Over time, I hope you find your sexual health voice and come to know what key content of each lesson is essential for a particular client population. This improvisational application of the curriculum is a creative opportunity that will develop only after a period of staying with the program. The saying "90 meetings in 90 days" is fundamentally based on the principle that repetition in early learning makes for a sound foundation for maintaining change over time.

I encourage you to gather a small team of sexual health experts, treatment experts, and group training experts to consult with during the first year of implementation. Many minds will make for good decisions as well as a better understanding of how to integrate sexual health with drug and alcohol treatment. I found that no one person has the combined training, skills, experience, and knowledge base to begin this program.

Must I Follow the Lessons in Order?

No. Each lesson is an independent experience. The lessons can be done in any order. A few of the lessons refer to skills or content from other lessons. This repetition is in the context of the current lesson and any questions that arise can be addressed in the current session. Lessons do not build upon content from previous lessons as a core component of learning. One caveat: each new person entering the program needs to complete the orientation session before beginning the 12-session sequence.

My goal was to structure the 12 lessons flexibly to accommodate the multiple acuity levels of drug and alcohol treatment. Some treatment centers may choose to include a limited number of sessions in their briefer inpatient programming. The entire program can also be offered as an outpatient service, a postintensive inpatient treatment follow-up, or a freestanding community program provided to anyone concerned about sex/drug-linked relapse.

In preparing this for publication, I had much ambivalence in numbering the lessons. It is so automatic to think we must go in order or that lesson number 1 is more important than lesson number 12. (In fact, Lesson 11, "Sexual Boundaries in Recovery," and Lesson 12, "Relationship With My Body," were consistent Stepping Stone client favorites.) I encourage you to experiment, be flexible, and be creative, but most of all be relevant to the need and circumstances of your treatment center. At Stepping Stone, the specific class could change on the very day depending on the overall tone and situations within the treatment program.

You will notice within the curriculum that no mention is made of the previous classes. This is to allow you the greatest flexibility in organizing the lessons. However, you may wish to refer back to previous classes, depending on client reaction and the treatment program. As you become more experienced, these creative clinical judgments will become easier.

What Is a Good Schedule for This Program?

The one place this program has been taught every week since 2003 is Stepping Stone in San Diego. Therefore, we don't have a lot of data to rely on regarding this question. Key elements of what I believe made the schedule so successful at Stepping Stone include the following.

The group met at a time when everyone in the program could and was required to attend. This program is not a pull out program for selected clients. Sexual health in recovery is essential for everyone. Some may need it more than others, but I believe that deciding that some people need this and others do not will create a sexual double standard. I believe one of the most important and crucial decisions Stepping Stone made was to make sexual health in recovery a basic element of their treatment. Every client was told upon his or her intake assessment that Stepping Stone was a sex-positive treatment program that integrated sexual health to improve treatment and reduce the risk of sex/drug-linked relapse *for every person in the treatment program*. Thus every client, regardless of his or her advancement in the treatment program, attended each session twice until he or she had completed 24 sessions. The community-based program and adult outpatient treatment program participants attended 12 or 24 sessions, depending on their preference.

Each group is 90 minutes from start to end. Starting and ending on time is basic good group work. Expect everyone to stay for the entire 90 minutes. There were several hundred participants in the grant evaluation period; only a handful had their entry into the group delayed because of unstable mental health or because the topic for that week was too stimulating for the first group. (Lesson 8, "Nonconsensual Sex," was the most common lesson to cause a 1-week delay.)

Schedule the groups so the group leader(s) have no responsibilities 30 minutes before and 30 minutes following the session. The details for preparation take time. Many participants have personal questions after class. Make sure there is time to reflect on what went well, make notes, put things away, and then breathe! Do not underestimate the level of work the first sequence will be. This curriculum is a stretch for many drug and alcoholism professionals. Like all endeavors, stick with it and you will be rewarded. Clients have been waiting for a program like this for a long time. The appreciation for leading this group and for attending to sex/drug-linked relapse with the refreshing news of sexual health is a gift you will be thanked for.

TALKING ABOUT SEX

A big unknown prior to beginning the sexual health in recovery program at Stepping Stone was how the clients and staff would respond to changes in the frequency and content of sexual conversations. The most significant change was the decrease in sexualized humor, sexualized distracting behavior between residents, and sexual tension regarding attractions and crushes between clients.

I believe that this is an outcome of a sexual health–based intervention. When a treatment center provides a sex-positive space to discuss sexual concerns related to sobriety from a sexual health perspective, it seems to diminish the pressure on other outlets that previously were the only space to discuss sex. Thus it is important for your treatment center to ask, "Where are our clients discussing sexuality now? With whom are they having these conversations?" The sexual health in recovery groups may quickly become the focal point for sexual matters in recovery to be addressed. This may free up clients to attend to other recovery concerns. For some men and women, it may be a significant relief to have a guaranteed treatment space for sex/drug-linked issues.

Talking about the wide range of sexual topics and interventions in this curriculum will expand most drug and alcohol counselors and treatment programs beyond their current level of comfort. An important growth for any sex educator is to invest in his or her own personal growth and professional knowledge regarding human sexuality.

There are several organizations that provide excellent training. One of the most useful experiences, in my opinion, it to attend a Sexual Attitude Reassessment seminar (SAR). A SAR is a process-oriented structured group experience to increase professionals' awareness of their attitudes and values and how these values affect their professional and personal life. A SAR is a basic prerequisite for becoming a certified sex therapist, counselor, or educator. SARs are offered through various organizations and conferences throughout the year. A schedule can be found at the American Association of Sexuality Educators, Counselors and Therapists (http://www.aasect.org).

As part of your preparation, it is important to be clear about terms and language that are unacceptable because they create an unsafe treatment environment. This is an important discussion to have before commencing the sexual health in recovery program. There are excellent resources online for leading sex education groups. I recommend visiting SexEd Library (http://www.sexedlibrary.org) and the "Professional

Development" section to learn more about leading a sexual education group in a safe and comfortable manner.

Finally, prior to beginning the curriculum, your program must determine how clients are expected to handle individual or private sexual concerns that emerge as a result of the sexual health in recovery group. For example, you may decide that high-risk sex/drug-linked clients be strongly encouraged to meet individually with a particular counselor to privately discuss his or her individual questions, concerns, treatment planning, as well as help with the worksheets from the lesson.

CORE CONCEPT

Being comfortable and willing to discuss sex and sexual matters in drug and alcohol treatment is an essential tool for beginning and maintaining recovery. Sexual health in drug and alcohol treatment is a cutting-edge intervention, one that is not taught yet at most drug treatment programs. Preliminary studies have concluded that clients whose drug use and sexual behavior go hand in hand—what we call sex/drug linked—will increase their chances of completing treatment and staying in recovery when they participate in a sexual health in recovery group.

BELIEF STATEMENT

Women and men in recovery increase their likelihood of staying sober when they complete a sexual health in drug and alcohol treatment program.

OBJECTIVES

Participants will
- Experience an interesting and affirming introduction to the content, logistics, and values of the sexual health in drug and alcohol treatment program.
- Become acquainted with the class facilitator(s).
- Increase comfort and familiarity with sexual health language and discussions.
- Learn treatment program sexual boundaries and guidelines.

■ Discuss their concerns, hopes, and goals for the sexual health in drug and alcohol treatment program.

CHANGE GOALS

■ Increase knowledge about the sexual health in drug and alcohol treatment program.
■ Increase motivation to participate in sexual health in drug and alcohol treatment program.
■ Learn expectations for sexual communication in the program.
■ Learn expectations for sexual behavior in the program.
■ Decrease discomfort and overwhelmed feelings with regard to sexual health information.

REQUIRED READING FOR GROUP LEADER

■ The Magnus Hirschfeld Archive for Sexology (www2.hu-berlin. de/sexology/index.htm) is the largest human sexuality Web site in the world. Currently available in 12 different languages, the Archive promotes sexual health by offering the best scientific information in one place on the Internet. For this class, leaders should familiarize themselves with the Critical Dictionary and Inappropriate Terms Dictionary. Reading the Inappropriate Terms Dictionary will provide excellent content for why certain sex terms are full of hidden value judgments, are imprecise, and are misleading. Compare the term in the Critical Dictionary to become familiar with language and definitions that are based on facts, research, and sex-positive perspectives.

RECOMMENDED MATERIALS FOR GROUP LEADER

■ Avert.org (www.avert.org/stories.htm) is a U.K. Web-based HIV prevention and sex education site. It features a personal story section about sex education experiences of youth. It provides an up-to-the-minute look at the strengths, weaknesses, and erroneous assumptions made by sex educators in the students own words. I find this content a humbling reminder of how difficult and yet how important sexual education experiences are, no matter what the age.

- Sex-Lexis.com (www.sex-lexis.com), is a Web-based independently, privately held online reference products company. It offers a location to input any of 24,150 sexual terms and expression from their Dictionary of Sex Words. For a group leader, this is an excellent source to refer to for any term, word, phrase, or sexological information a group member asks and you do not have the answer.

REQUIRED MATERIALS FOR THE LESSON

- An mp3 player and music selection
- Blackboard, white board, or flip chart
- Large posters labeled with scientific sexual terms (see the "Lecture" section for a suggested list of terms)
- Colored markers for participants
- Group schedule (one copy for each participant)

OPENING

Opening Music: Have quiet music playing as participants enter the room and ready themselves (optional).

Leader: As we sit quietly and focus on being here, let us clear our minds of where we have been and focus on being in this moment.

Opening Poem/Reading:

It takes courage to push yourself to places that you have never been before . . . to test your limits . . . to break through barriers. And the day came when the risk it took to remain tight inside the bud was more painful than the risk it took to blossom.

—Anaïs Nin

GROUP INTRODUCTION

Leader reads the following introduction:

Welcome to the sexual health in recovery group. We are here to talk about sex and how a our sexual lives affect recovery from drug and alcohol addiction. Some people in recovery risk a relapse because of their sexual behavior at the treatment center or away from the treatment program. This is a place to talk about sexual behavior and sexual health so we can be abstinent from drugs and alcohol. It is also a place to learn about sexual behavior and situations that put men and women in recovery at risk for not completing this treatment program.

Sexual health in recovery is a time to talk about human sexuality and sexual health in a respectful and informed manner. We encourage everyone to be as honest and open as you can be. You are not required to reveal anything about your current or past sexual behavior that would be uncomfortable to discuss. It is important to listen to each other. For some of us, our sexual behavior is the most serious risk to staying in recovery. For others, our sexual behavior gets us into dangerous situations that are triggers to use or drink. A few of us may have little concern about how our sexual behavior contributes to relapse. This group is an opportunity for everyone to learn about the important connection between recovery and sexual health.

LECTURE

Leader: Welcome to the orientation session for sexual health in drug and alcohol treatment. The goal of this program is to reduce relapse among men and women in recovery by addressing their sexual behavior patterns that may be linked with drinking and/or using drugs. Every client at this treatment program will attend this program. It is important to provide you with an opportunity to learn about the program, what is expected of you as you participate in the classes, as well as some fun to prepare you for entering an environment focused on sexual health.

Leader(s) take a few moments to introduce themselves, say a few words about their job, and perhaps a few words about why they are interested in working in this field.

Leader: The goals for today are to provide an introduction to the content, logistics and values of the sexual health in drug and alcohol treatment program. We will do some exercises that will provide opportunities to become more familiar with sexual health language and conversations. We will review client sexual behavior guidelines and expectations while in treatment. We want you to discuss any concerns and questions you may have about participating in the program. An educational group focused on sexual health is a very rare experience for most adults. We hope this orientation group makes beginning the sexual health in recovery group a more relaxed experience.

Leader: Before we get into the specifics of the program, let's start by discussing each of our individual experiences and history with sex education. Let's make a list on the board of the various places we may learn about sex, reproduction, sexuality, sexual orientation, sexual values, sexual ethics, sexual turn-ons, sexual abuse, sexual trauma, sexual crimes, or sexual relationships.

Write participants' responses on the board; do not edit or critique responses. Common responses may be friends, Internet, movies, parents' sex videos, parents' sex talk, siblings, relative, school sex education class, church sex education, television, music videos, and so forth.

This is the first time that group members will be participating in the group, so letting their experience be acknowledged will model an openness and receptiveness for participation. Try to give each member of the group at least one opportunity to contribute to the list.

Leader: Now let's circle the sex education experiences that you think were helpful and useful.

Again, take comments in an open manner that welcomes participants' comments.

Leader: As you think about the sex education experiences that were helpful, what was it that you experienced in these situations that made them useful and helpful?

Facilitate a brief discussion (no more than 5 minutes) among members about their positive experiences with sex education. Common responses usually revolve around feeling safe, not feeling embarrassed, feeling that they could ask questions without embarrassment, that the person providing information was calm and confident, that they were not overwhelmed with too much information, that the person was respectful and nonjudgmental, and that the information was useful.

Leader: Throughout your experience in the sexual health in recovery program we hope you will give feedback about what is helpful and useful as well as what concerns you. Because this is such a new service, your experiences will be valuable in developing and continually improving what we are trying to do.

Leader: The purpose for this orientation class is to make sure you are prepared to learn about sexual health in recovery. In order to learn about sexual health, we must increase our comfort with having sexually focused conversations. Today we are going to have an experience of writing and saying various sexual terms out loud together.

We want you to be prepared to enter the sexual health in recovery group classes. The first sexual health skill we want to teach is more effective and accurate sexual language. We are going to focus on language related to body parts and areas that are the usual sexual zones on our body. One of the most common barriers in discussing sexuality is the actual terms we use for discussing body parts, types of sexual activity, and sexual orientation. To increase our familiarity with all the different words used to describe sexuality we will spend some time having some fun as well as getting more comfortable with talking about sex with each other.

Why do you think sexual words, especially words about our genitals or areas of our body that are pleasurable to have touched or to touch on someone else are so uncomfortable to say?

Lead a brief discussion on thoughts and ideas participants have about sexual talk.

Leader: Why do you think sexual terms and language may be uncomfortable to discuss here at the treatment program?

Lead a brief discussion on thoughts and ideas participants have about sexual talk at the drug treatment program.

Leader: We are going to do a class exercise to assist people in expanding their sexual health language and to help reduce the giggle or tough guy effect in talking about sex. The giggle effect is the nervous laughter we automatically feel when we are doing something we feel a bit nervous, a bit excited, a bit daring, and a bit vulnerable doing. The tough guy effect is making sure everyone knows you do not need this sex ed stuff. For some of us, acknowledging not knowing something, especially about sex, risks being humiliated, made fun of, or even risks danger. This class is designed to provide you with some practice in getting past these reactions so you can learn about sexual health in recovery. We want you to have as much fun and laughter about sexual terms and language today so that when you are in the group sessions you can focus on things other than your discomfort about saying or listening to sex talk. So today, giggles, laughing, and having fun are expected and will be part of our learning.

Pin up the posters with familiar scientific sexual terms around the room. (Terms can include: breasts, clitoris, vagina, penis, testicles, buttocks, anus, intercourse, oral sex, masturbation, heterosexual, bisexual, and homosexual.) Place colored markers near each sheet.

Leader: Now I want each of you to pick up a marker and write appropriate slang terms for the scientific terms that you see on each sheet.

Allow participants time to quickly circulate and write on each sheet.

Leader: OK, now let's look over the lists and read them aloud together. That's right, let's read them in unison, saying each word out loud together.

Lead the group in unison, reading each word on the first list and moving on to the next. Keep going until everyone has read all the lists aloud together.

Leader: What are people feeling after this exercise?

Lead a discussion about reactions during the exercise. Invite each person in the group to share a brief comment. This is an important time for establishing a group norm of encouraging everyone to participate. If someone has no comment, offer a welcoming response and move on. The important issue is that the participants know you are aware of their presence without imposing participation.

Leader: When is the use of sexual slang appropriate? Which of the slang terms the group has listed are positive and which ones are derogatory?

Lead a discussion asking these questions and facilitating group interaction. Keep the group focused on answering the questions and staying focused on the exercise.

Leader: What language is appropriate here at the treatment program? What terms would make sexual discussion in class or around the treatment program feel unsafe or disrespectful?

Lead a discussion asking these questions and facilitating group interaction. As part of your preparation, you should be clear about terms and language that are unacceptable because they create an unsafe treatment environment.

Leader: When we feel unsafe or disrespected because of sexual slang or language, it may be a signal that a personal boundary is being crossed. Everyone has boundaries about sex. They vary greatly from person to person and from situation to situation. For example, a small peck on the lips may be a common way for family or close friends to greet, but it would be a boundary crossing if someone pecks you on the lips when he or she is meeting you for the first time. One of the goals for the sexual behavior relapse prevention program is to assist people in recovery to maintain respectful sexual boundaries. Let's talk for a few minutes about your current understanding of respectful sexual boundaries in treatment.

Invite participants to review the rules, policies, expectations, and boundaries about sexual behavior that are in place in your treatment facility. Topics may include having sex with other clients, masturbation, having sex with other members of Alcoholics Anonymous/Narcotics Anonymous, flirtatious behavior, nudity, sex with roommates, and so forth. Write each example on the board.

Leader: That looks like a pretty good list. Let's talk for a few minutes about how these boundaries are about respect and safety for everyone who is in treatment.

Invite discussion that focuses on safety and respect rather than only following the rules. Try to get participants to see how crossing boundaries may increase a feeling of disrespect or lack of safety.

Leader: Some sexual boundary violations are significant mistakes because they may be unsafe or even illegal, for example, forcing someone to have sex or using extortion to have sex with someone (e.g., if you don't have sex with me I will do something to hurt or endanger you). Other sexual boundary crossings are mistakes that require a significant response by the counseling staff. The response is necessary because your sexual mistake may risk your own sobriety or the sobriety of other clients. What are some examples of sexual mistakes that you think could risk your own sobriety or the sobriety of others?

Lead a discussion of examples of sexual mistakes that may be linked with risk for using drugs/alcohol.

Leader: The sexual health in drug and alcohol treatment program is here to help everyone respond to residents' sexual mistakes in a responsible and thoughtful manner. Women and men in recovery are learning to live a full and complete life. As Stephanie Covington, a noted expert in sexuality and recovery says: "Sexual recovery is not a calm ocean that you sail over like a stately ocean liner. You will still have your ups and down. But in recovery, as opposed to addiction, you have hope. You know that you can change your sexual patterns, because you already have. The hopelessness of addiction is no longer your constant state of being. And as you gain hope, you also begin to gain personal power" (Covington, 2000, p. 145).

The sexual health in recovery program is here to assess, educate, and support your sexual lives throughout your treatment. Risk for relapse will decrease when clients are provided a safe place to discuss sexual concerns. Too many men and women fail to complete treatment or relapse in their recovery when they do not have a place to address sexual concerns and worries. Sexual health in recovery is the place to learn, discuss, ask questions, listen, and practice how to address sexuality in recovery.

Now we will take a few moments to look at the various components of this program. The program will include a 12-session educational group that meets every week for 90 minutes. Every client at this treatment center is required to attend each of the 12 sessions. The sexual health in recovery meetings will be an educational class. Each class will be lead by me (or if co-leaders, by us). Some of the meetings will separate into smaller groups for discussion. Each class will revolve around four general themes:

1. The sex/drug link
2. Sexual attitudes and values
3. Sexual history
4. Sexual health

Leader: I am handing out a complete roster of the program with the dates for each group outlined. This schedule will be updated as needed.

Hand out the group schedule.

Leader: Group will begin and end on time. Each class will include a combination of information, experiential exercises, and in-class practice of sexual health recovery tools. At the end of each session, you will be given a worksheet to take with you and practice throughout your recovery.

> *Review the 12 classes, discuss each title, respond to questions or concerns about the classes.*
> *Provide direction for how your program has determined where clients should take individual or private sexual concerns emerging as a result of the sexual health in recovery group. For example, you may say that the program also includes opportunities to meet individually with a particular counselor and that clients can schedule appointments to privately discuss individual questions, concerns, treatment planning, as well as help with the worksheets that will be handed out in the group.*

Leader: Before we close this orientation group, let's take a few moments to talk about your reactions, thoughts, or comments about entering into this program as part of your overall treatment. What reactions or comments do you have?

> *Welcome comments, correct misunderstandings, clarify any misinformation; encourage individuals to schedule individual appointments if significant individual concerns are raised that cannot be addressed in the orientation session.*

Leader: Is there anything else to discuss before we bring our meeting to a close?

EXPERIENTIAL LEARNING

None.

TOPIC SKILL PRACTICE

None.

CLOSING

Leader: Now let's take a moment to bring the workshop to a close. Let's take a moment to take a deep breath and quiet our mind, our hearts, and our spirit. In this quiet place, remind yourself how valuable it is to take the time to be honest, vulnerable, and committed to recovery. As you leave the group today, remind yourself that a satisfying sexual life is a vital and important part of recovery. The self-reflection and tools you learned today may become an important part of maintaining your recovery.

REFERENCES

Avert.org. (2009). Retrieved from www.avert.org.

Covington, S. (2000). *Awakening your sexuality: A guide for recovering women.* Center City, MN: Hazelden.

Nin, Anaïs. (2009). *Quotes on courage.* About Personal Growth, Malaysia. Retrieved May 24, 2009, from www.about-personal-growth.com/quotes-on-courage.html

Sex-Lexis.com. (2004). Retrieved from sex-lexis.com.

Sex/Drug-Linked Sexual Health

Sex/Drug-Linked Relapse Risk

CORE CONCEPT

Too many clients prematurely terminate drug and alcohol treatment and eventually relapse. Men and women who successfully complete a drug and alcohol treatment program drastically reduce their risk for relapse. Sexual health in recovery believes that the link between drug and alcohol use and sex can be a central reason for failing to complete treatment and relapse. When drug and alcohol treatment educates recovering addicts about the link between sex and using, treatment outcomes improve. An important sex/drug-linked recovery skill is thinking through which sexual situations are risky for relapse. In this session, participants examine sexual situations linked with their relapse risk and practice utilizing the "Stopping and Thinking About Sex/Drug Situations in Recovery Worksheet" (Lesson 1 appendix).

BELIEF STATEMENT

Sexual health in recovery is the ability to connect sexual situations with level of risk for relapse.

OBJECTIVES

Participants will
- Learn common sex/drug-linked situations connected with increasing risk for relapse.
- Practice rating levels of relapse risk with other women and men in drug and alcohol treatment.
- Learn the stop and think recovery skill for responding to sexual situations during and following treatment.
- Practice essential self-reflection skills before entering sexual situations.

CHANGE GOALS

- Normalize necessity to consider relapse risk as part of sexual life in recovery.
- Increase skills in self-reflection prior to entering sexual situations.
- Increase skills in critically evaluating sex/drug-linked relapse risk in sexual situations.

REQUIRED READING FOR GROUP LEADER

Marlatt, A., & Donovan, D. (Eds.) (2005). *Relapse prevention: Maintenance strategies in the treatment of addictive behaviors*. New York: Guilford Press.

Chapter 5 ("Relapse Prevention for Stimulant Dependence") by Carroll and Rawson and Chapter 8 ("Relapse Prevention for Abuse of Club Drugs, Hallucinogens, Inhalants, and Steroids") by Kilmer, Cronce, and Palmer provide an excellent overview of the high frequency sex-linked drugs. The confluence of sex/drug-linked relapse risk is not a concept specifically reviewed in either chapter. Sexual health is not addressed as a concept for treatment or relapse prevention. Shame is not addressed directly as a relapse risk factor.

That said, reading these two chapters will confirm many elements of the leadership style, format, experiential group learning, and cognitive-behavioral elements of the sexual health in recovery curriculum. "In some instances it will be necessary to illustrate for the client the ways in which substance use may be impacting other problems in his or her life, particularly if the individual is passionate about addressing a particular problem in therapy and is reluctant to make changes in substance use" (Kilmer, Cronce, & Palmer, 2005, p. 229).

> Once other treatment needs of the client are identified, these too can become a focus of therapy, particularly if their continued existence serves as a high-risk situation for an individual. As an example, steroid users find that decreased sexual function can occur following cessation of use. Addressing this, therefore, will be of utmost importance if problems with sexual functioning lead to resuming use. (Kilmer et al., 2005, p. 230)

RECOMMENDED MATERIALS FOR GROUP LEADER

I recommend the following materials, which focus on key elements of sex/drug-linked behavior. The research literature often focuses on crystal methamphetamine sex/drug-linked behavior and consequences for HIV infection, HIV transmission to uninfected partners, and other sexually transmitted infections (STIs). Sex/drug-linked issues that focus on men who have sex with male partners or who identify as gay are most widely found in stimulant abuse or addiction research.

- *Tweakers: How Crystal Meth Is Ravaging Gay America,* by Frank Sanello. (2005). Los Angeles: Alyson Publications. (Chapter 6, "Dating Tina: Sex on Meth," pp. 123–145, is an excellent review of sex/drug-linked motivations for meth and sex,).
- *Crystal Meth and Men Who Have Sex With Men: What Mental Health Care Professionals Need to Know,* edited by Milton Wainberg, Andrew Kolodny, and Jack Drescher. (2006). Binghamton, NY: The Haworth Medical Press. (In "HIV Risk Behaviors Among Gay Male Methamphetamine Users: Before and After Treatment," Sherry Larkins, Cathy Reback, and Steven Shoptaw write that "addressing both the methamphetamine use and its associated high-risk sex are of paramount importance when treating an addiction that is so intertwined with sexual behavior" (2006, p. 125).
- The 2007 National Institute on Drug Abuse (NIDA) Science Meeting "Drug Abuse and Risky Behaviors: The Evolving Dynamics of HIV/AIDS" included a paper by Denise Hallfors titled, "Do Sex and Drug Behavior Patterns Account for HIV/

STD Racial Disparities?" In the paper, Hallfors identifies 11 risk behavior patterns that were correlated with increased risk for STI/HIV infection among non-Hispanic Blacks compared with Whites. In summary, she found that among U.S. White young adults STI/HIV infection risk is elevated only when associated with high-risk behavior. Black young adults remained at high STI/HIV infection risk even if their behavior is normative. The African American young adult women in the study were the least likely to engage in alcohol, tobacco, and other drug use behaviors but the most likely to acquire STIs. Hallfors suggested two contextual factors that may account for this difference. One factor is the more frequent sexual crossover between high-risk males and low-risk females within African American young adult women compared to White young adults. Second is the correlation between high school dropout, poverty, and early sexual debut.

■ At the same 2007 NIDA meeting, Gail Wyatt, PhD presented a paper titled, "How Does Trauma Contribute to Substance Abuse and HIV Infection Among Ethnic Women?" Wyatt identifies seven distinguishing HIV infection risk factors among African American women. Many of these factors are sex-linked risks that are addressed in sexual health in recovery (i.e., sexual health, relationships, trauma, perceived worth [shame]). The Wyatt and Hallfors studies both point to the importance of tailoring sex/drug-linked interventions within gender and cultural factors.

■ *Meth* (Ahlberg, 2005) is a documentary film in which current and past gay male meth users are shown with honesty and candor. The film leaves the viewer profoundly sad and informed about the significance of the sex/drug link in crystal methamphetamine addiction. The trailer and DVD ordering information is at http://www.methmovie.com or contact the director Todd Ahlberg at Babalu Pictures (todd@babalupictures.com).

■ Knowcrystal.org is a multimedia San Diego–based Web site for gay and bisexual men contemplating their current use of crystal meth. Knowcrystal.org provides a range of factual information on the impact of methamphetamine in a judgment-free environment. This is not a site for men in recovery. I recommend it for counselors to increase their understanding of sex/drug-linked sexual behavior. It provides innovative sexual health approaches, including a range of resources and information targeting users, those who may be at-risk for using, as well as resources for family and friends of gay and bisexual crystal using men.

REQUIRED MATERIALS FOR THE LESSON

- An mp3 player and music selection
- Blackboard, white board, or flip chart
- Numbered index cards, labeled 0–10 (one set for each participant)
- "Stopping and Thinking About Sex/Drug Situations in Recovery Worksheet" (one copy for each participant) (Lesson 1 appendix)

OPENING

Opening Music: *Have quiet music playing as participants enter the room and ready themselves (optional).*

Leader: As we sit quietly and focus on being here, let us clear our minds of where we have been and focus on being in this moment.

Opening Poem/Reading:

Sobriety is an astonishing, revelatory, wonderful gift; few recovering alcoholics and drug addicts who've managed to stay sober for any length of time would disagree with this. But despite our newfound clarity, few of us escape having problems with sex, intimacy, and love. . . . We experience some of our greatest blocks in the sexual arena because, for most of us, sex requires a degree of nakedness (psychic as well as physical) that few recovering people are willing to experience without the buffering, muting, fantasizing effects of drugs and alcohol

—G. Kettelhack, *How to Make Love While Conscious* (1993)

GROUP INTRODUCTION

Have a group member volunteer to read aloud.

Welcome to the sexual health in recovery group. We are here to talk about sex and how our sexual lives affect recovery from drug and alcohol addiction. Some people in recovery risk a relapse because of their sexual behavior at the treatment center or away from the treatment program. This is a place to talk about sexual behavior and sexual health so we can be abstinent from drugs and alcohol. It is also a place to learn about sexual behavior and situations that put men and women in recovery at risk for not completing this treatment program.

Sexual health in recovery is a time to talk about human sexuality and sexual health in a respectful and informed manner. We encourage everyone to be as honest and open as you can be. You are not required to reveal anything about your current or past sexual behavior that would be uncomfortable to discuss. It is important to listen to each other. For some of us, our sexual behavior is the most serious risk to staying in recovery. For others, our sexual behavior gets us into dangerous situations that are triggers to use or drink. A few of us may have little concern about how our sexual behavior contributes to relapse. This group is an opportunity for everyone to learn about the important connection between recovery and sexual health.

LESSON INTRODUCTION

Ask another group member to volunteer to read aloud.

The purpose of today's sexual health in recovery group is to discuss the link between recovery from alcoholism and/or drug addiction and sexual behavior.

We believe that women and men in recovery increase their likelihood of staying sober when they connect sexual situations with level of risk for relapse. Recovery will increase if the sexual situations linked with getting high are anticipated and thought through. Recovering people need to learn how to stop and think before entering unfamiliar sober sexual situations. Today we will talk about sexual situations and circumstances that are commonly linked with drinking and drugs. We will learn to rate the level of relapse risk in both our past and current sexual situations. We will discuss the value of stopping and thinking, taking time to pause and reflect about sex/drug relapse risk before entering high-risk sexual situations. Taking time to think before getting into sexual situations is an essential skill in recovery. We will learn how to use the "Stopping and Thinking About Sex/Drug Situations in Recovery Worksheet" and practice using this recovery tool in the group.

LECTURE

Leader: Today we are going to talk about our sexual behavior, thoughts, and decisions that may be closely linked with using drugs or alcohol. Many of you have probably been in situations where you were using alcohol and/or drugs as part of your sexual behavior. You may have used drugs to try something new sexually. You may have gotten drunk or high to just feel sexual or to do something that you might be too embarrassed or anxious to do sober. You may have gotten high to feel more in love or connected with your partner. You may have gotten high in order to tolerate or forget a terrible sexual experience. You probably had many different circumstances for being high before, during, or after sex.

We will begin the session with discussing why addressing sexual behavior linked with addiction is so important. New information suggests people have better treatment outcomes when their sexual relationships and behavior linked with drug use are directly addressed in all phases of recovery. Some people with a very high level of sex/drug-linked behavior will not remain sober without skills to prevent relapse in sexual situations. Traditionally, alcohol and drug recovery centers have relegated addressing sexual behavior in early recovery to the back burner or have believed that to address sexuality too soon in recovery risks client relapse or termination from treatment. Conversations about sex are even taboo in some alcohol and drug treatment centers; even members of the staff have a difficult time broaching the subject.

Today we are going to focus on two aspects of sex/drug-linked relapse. First, we will look at past sexual situations and how often drugs/alcohol were linked. We will then look at how to predict the likelihood of risk for using in future sexual situations.

These are the five general motivations for sex/drug linked behavior:

1. To increase ability to sexually function (e.g., to make an erection last longer or not lose an erection, to increase control about when you orgasm or ejaculate, to increase ability to have intercourse, to have a more intense orgasm, to delay orgasm, to bring your partner to orgasm).
2. To change level of sexual interest, desire, or arousal (e.g., having low interest in sex, only feeling sexually turned on when high, inability to have sex without being high, frequency of sexual desire, too much sexual desire, too little sexual desire, wanting to have an orgasm, wanting to give your partner pleasure).

3. To experience a specific sexual turn-on. Using drugs or alcohol to perform a specific sex act (e.g., feeling embarrassed about sexual desires that are supposedly strange or perverted, having specific fetish activities, having same-sex desires, desiring specific sexual acts like oral sex, anal sex, oral–anal sex, sex without a condom, or various unconventional turn-ons).

4. To escape from negative or overwhelming feelings. Using sex to get out of a negative or overwhelming feeling and to experience sexual pleasure or excitement instead (e.g., wanting to escape from coming down, wanting to escape from the overwhelming consequences of drug use, feeling less ugly or unwanted, being afraid to have sex sober, feeling worried your spouse or partner is going to leave you, wanting to end your marriage or relationship).

5. To express feelings of love, affection, and commitment. Using drugs and alcohol to express love to a partner or to receive expressions of love from a partner. (For example, wanting to feel close, wanting to feel loved, needing to be touched, wanting to feel comforted, wanting to express my love for my partner).

EXPERIENTIAL LEARNING

Leader: Raise your hand if you have ever been asked to rate something about yourself using the numbers 1 to 10. As you can see, this is a very common way to self-reflect and measure something about ourselves. We are going to do an exercise where we will do a group self-reflection using a scale with numbers between 0 and 10.

Draw a line on the board with numbers 0–10 on a continuum:

0   1   2   3   4   5   6   7   8   9   10

Leader: I am going to label the numbers on each end with the words "Never" and "Always." Zero means that something never applies to you; 10 means you cannot think of even one time this did *not* apply to you.

Label each end of the continuum with extreme positions on sex/drug-linked behavior:

0   1   2   3   4   5   6   7   8   9   10
Never   Always

Leader: What we are going to rate is how often your were motivated to use sex and drugs together for a specific circumstance. We will use the examples from the five general motivations that we discussed just a moment ago. You will each have a numbered deck of cards.

Hand out decks of numbered cards (0–10) to each participant.

Leader: Each card has a number 0 through 10. I will ask a group member to briefly describe a sex/drug-linked situation from our list. Listen to the description and choose a number between 0 and 10 that rates how often this particular situation was a motivator for you to combine sex and drugs before entering treatment. After everyone has chosen a number I will ask everyone to hold their card up so I can write all the numbers on the continuum. We will repeat this several times.

> *Have a member of the group describe a sex/drug-linked situation from one of the categories above. Ask participants to rate themselves on a scale of 0–10 according to how often this particular situation was part of their sex/drug-linked behavior before entering treatment. Have everyone raise their cards. Tally the numbers. Write the range of answers on the board to show the range of "Never" to "Always" responses within the class.*
>
> *Repeat several times (do at least one situation from each of the five categories). Facilitate a brief group discussion of the reasons why drugs or alcohol may be linked with these situations. Discuss gender differences in sex/drug-linked motivations and situations. Current research shows significant differences between men and women in their responses to sexual situations (Bancroft, Graham, Janssen, & Sanders, 2009; Chivers, Rieger, Latty, & Baily, 2004; Janssen & Bancroft, 2006).*

Leader: We will see throughout the various sexual health in recovery lessons how men and women differ in their responses to sexual situations. It will be the job of everyone to be curious and interested in these gender differences as they are discussed in the sessions.

Take a few minutes to have participants share how it felt to do this exercise.

Leader: Now we are going to move from focusing on past sex/drug-linked situations to current sexual situations in recovery that are linked with drugs and alcohol.

Draw another line on the board with numbers 0–10 on a continuum.

0	1	2	3	4	5	6	7	8	9	10

Not at all likely   Very likely

Leader: Now we will review the five sex/drug-linked situations from the perspective of being in recovery.

Review the list again and begin the discussion.
    Have a group member describe a sexual situation in recovery from one of the five categories. Using the deck of numbered cards, ask participants to evaluate how likely a person currently in drug/alcohol treatment will remain sober in this particular sexual situation. Have everyone raise their card and record the answers on the white board continuum to show the range of "Not at all likely" to "Very likely" within the class.
    Repeat several times and facilitate a discussion. Do at least one situation from each of the five categories. Facilitate a brief group discussion of the reasons why these may be low or high likelihood of remaining sober.

TOPIC SKILL PRACTICE

Leader: We just practiced the skill we are going to teach today: to pause and think about a sexual situation in regard to staying sober. The purpose of this exercise is to allow time to think about the relapse risk in sexual situations prior to taking action. "Thinking before doing" is the message. Recovery requires taking a few moments to reflect before taking action. Thinking about our sexual desires and pausing to reflect on our motives is an important relapse prevention tool for sexual health in recovery.

Leader: Today we are going to learn and practice a specific tool to connect sexual situations with risk for using drugs and alcohol. This tool is a worksheet that provides a space to think about risk of relapse before taking action in any sexual situation in recovery. This skill is especially useful for behaviors that have become so habitual in our drug use that it is almost like they are a reflex—we do them without having to think. For sexual health in recovery, taking a few moments to reflect before taking action is a very important recovery tool.

Hand out the "Stopping and Thinking About Sex/Drug Situations in Recovery Worksheet" (Lesson 1 appendix).

Leader: We are going to do a practice exercise to demonstrate how to use this worksheet. The first task is to describe a sexual situation or circumstance that may come up while in treatment. For example, someone makes a pass at you at a 12-step meeting. You are riding the bus and see a very attractive person that reminds you of a person you would have sex with and get high. Your spouse liked sex better when you were both high. You are only attracted to people for a short fling. Who would like to volunteer to practice using this exercise?

Choose a volunteer to come to the front of the group.

Leader: To begin the exercise, tell us a sexual situation or behavior that may come up while in treatment. You do not need to personally disclose if this situation is real for you right now. We will not assume we know why you have chosen to describe the situation you are telling us about. Now write the sexual situation on the board as you would write it on the worksheet.

Allow time for the volunteer to write a situation on the board.

Leader: Now let's think about which of the five sex/drug-linked situations exist in this scenario.

Lead a brief discussion of what other members of the group think.

Leader: Now stop and think for a moment and then rate how likely this sexual situation or behavior will increase your risk for relapse.

Volunteer rates the situation. Ask the remainder of class to silently choose from their numbered cards how likely of a relapse risk the situation would be for them.

Leader: Stop and think and then rate how likely this sexual situation or behavior will increase your likelihood of staying sober.

Volunteer rates the situation. Ask the remainder of class to silently choose from their numbered cards to rate how likely this sexual situation or behavior will increase their likelihood of staying sober.
Have the volunteer look at his or her answers and then think aloud with the group why they might or might not still consider this sexual activity.

Leader: This is an exercise you all can do at any time in your recovery. Let's talk for a few minutes about when this worksheet may be useful while in treatment. How might it be a recovery tool after completing treatment? Stopping and thinking about our sexual behavior and the impact it may have on our recovery is an important skill for enjoying sex and evaluating risk for relapse.

CLOSING

Leader: Now let's take a moment to bring the workshop to a close. Let's take a moment to again quiet ourselves, take a deep breath to quiet our minds, our hearts, and our spirits. In this quiet place, remind yourself how valuable it is to take the time to be honest, vulnerable, and committed to recovery. As you leave the group today, remind yourself that a satisfying sexual life is a vital and important part of recovery. The self-reflection and tools you learned today may become an important part of maintaining your recovery.

REFERENCES

Ahlberg, T. (2005). *Meth* [Motion picture]. United States: Babalu Pictures.

Bancroft, J., Graham, C., Janssen, E., & Sanders, S. (2009). The dual control model: Current status and future directions. *Journal of sex research, 46*(2–3), 121–142.

Carroll, K., & Rawson, R. (2005). Relapse prevention for stimulant dependence. In A. Marlatt, & D. Donovan (Eds.), *Relapse prevention: Maintenance strategies in the treatment of addictive behaviors* (pp. 130–150). New York: Guilford Press.

Chivers, M., Rieger, G., Latty, E., & Baily, M. (2004). A sex difference in the specificity of sexual arousal. *Psychological Science, 15*(11), 736–744.

Hallfors, D. (2007, May). *Do sex and drug behavior patterns account for HIV/STD racial disparities?* Paper presented at the National Institute on Drug Abuse Science Meeting, Bethesda, Maryland.

Janssen, E., & Bancroft, J. (2006). The dual control model: The role of sexual inhibition and excitation in sexual arousal and behavior. In E. Janssen, (Ed.), *The psychophysiology of sex*. Bloomington: Indiana University Press.

Kettelhack, G. (1993). *How to make love while conscious: Sex and sobriety*. New York: HarperCollins.

Kilmer, J., Cronce, J., & Palmer, R. (2005). Relapse prevention for abuse of club drugs, hallucinogens, inhalants, and steroids. In A. Marlatt & D. Donovan (Eds.), *Relapse prevention: Maintenance strategies in the treatment of addictive behaviors* (pp. 208–247). New York: Guilford Press.

Larkins, S., Reback, C., & Shoptaw, S. (2006). HIV risk behaviors among gay male methamphetamine users: Before and after treatment. In M. Wainberg, A. Kolodny, &

J. Drescher (Eds.), *Crystal meth and men who have sex with men: What mental health care professionals need to know* (pp. 123–129). Binghamton, NY: The Haworth Medical Press.

Marlatt, A., & Donovan, D. (Eds.) (2005). *Relapse prevention: Maintenance strategies in the treatment of addictive behaviors.* New York: Guilford Press.

Sanello, F. (2005). *Tweakers: How crystal meth is ravaging gay America.* Los Angeles: Alyson Publications.

Wainberg, M., Kolodny, A., & Drescher, J. (Eds.) (2006). *Crystal meth and men who have sex with men: What mental health care professionals need to know.* Binghamton, NY: The Haworth Medical Press.

Wyatt, G. (2007, May). *How does trauma contribute to substance abuse and HIV infection among ethnic women?* Paper presented at the National Institute on Drug Abuse Science Meeting, Bethesda, Maryland.

LESSON 1 APPENDIX

Stopping and Thinking About Sex/Drug Situations in Recovery Worksheet

What sexual situation or behavior do I need to stop and think about?

_____

_____

_____

Put a Check Mark Next to Each Sex/Drug-Linked Motivation in This Specific Sexual Situation

_____ Increase ability to sexually function. Using drugs or alcohol to sexually function.

_____ Change level of sexual interest, desire, or arousal. Using drugs or alcohol to feel interested in sex.

_____ Experience a specific sexual turn-on. Using drugs or alcohol to perform a specific sex act or an unusual or kinky sex act.

_____ Escape from negative or overwhelming feelings. Using sex to get out of a negative or overwhelming feeling and to experience sexual pleasure or excitement instead.

_____ Express feelings of love, affection, and commitment. Using drugs and alcohol to express love to a partner or to receive expressions of love from a partner.

Stop and think for a moment and then rate how often this sexual situation or behavior was linked with using drugs or drinking before recovery:

    0   1   2   3   4   5   6   7   8   9   10

Never   Always

Stop and think for a moment and then rate how likely this sexual situation or behavior will increase your risk for relapse:

| 0 | 1 | 2 | 3 | 4 | 5 | 6 | 7 | 8 | 9 | 10 |

Not at all likely   Very likely

Stop and think for a moment and then rate how likely this sexual situation or behavior will increase your likelihood of staying sober:

| 0 | 1 | 2 | 3 | 4 | 5 | 6 | 7 | 8 | 9 | 10 |

Not at all likely   Very likely

Read the specific sex/drug-linked situation again. Review the motivations you checked. Review the three ratings. Pause and think for a moment. Now write an answer to the question: Why am I still motivated to pursue this sexual activity?

_____

_____

_____

2   Sexual Decisions in Recovery

CORE CONCEPT

Women and men in early recovery may be ready to stop using drugs and drinking but lack interest in changing anything about their sexual behavior. This conflict between the willingness to treat addiction and readiness to address sexual behavior (even when sex may risk relapse or treatment failure) is the focus of this class. Experts in the process of change discovered that when people understand how their attitudes and defenses are obstructing their process of change, their resistance to change is reduced. Sexual decisions in recovery improve when men and women in treatment understand how defenses may interfere with thinking about sex/drug-linked situations. The "Common Defenses That Interfere With Knowing How Sexual Life Impacts Recovery" handout and the "Sexual Behavior Consciousness Raising Self-Assessment" worksheet (Lesson 2 appendix, A and B) are tools to increase self-honesty and awareness of defenses that interfere with talking about sex. Participants will measure their readiness to look more honestly at sexual situations and their ability to look at their sex/drug-linked relapse risk.

BELIEF STATEMENT

Sexual health in recovery is the ability to honestly self reflect in sexual decisions regarding relapse risk level.

OBJECTIVES

Participants will
- Assess thoughts and feelings about commonly held sexual attitudes and advice for early recovery.
- Learn common defense mechanisms that interfere with self-reflection about changing sexual decision making.
- Assess and measure readiness for changing sexual decisions that reduce relapse risk.

CHANGE GOALS

- Increase knowledge about using consciousness-raising tools for contemplating sexual decisions.
- Utilize consciousness-raising assessment tools for contemplating sexual decisions before taking action.
- Increase ability for honest self-reflection about sexual desires that may contribute to relapse.

REQUIRED READING FOR GROUP LEADER

- *Changing for Good: A Revolutionary Six-Stage Program for Overcoming Bad Habits and Moving Your Life Positively Forward,* by Prochaska, Norcross, and DiClemente (1994). This book teaches the general public about the stages of change process. Chapter 4, "Precontemplation—Resisting Change," (pp. 73–108) is the source material for this curriculum. The authors outline seven high-frequency defenses of precontemplators. The group leader should be very conversant about how these defenses "distract us from the difficult and uncomfortable task of self-analysis" (p. 82).

The "Common Defenses That Interfere With Knowing How Sexual Life Impacts Recovery" handout and the "Sexual Behavior Consciousness Raising Self-Assessment" are adaptations of the self-assessment measures from this chapter. A key concept when beginning to address sex/drug-linked relapse risk is to recognize our defenses without the implicit demand to stop being defensive. Being able to observe defenses (without requiring the elimination of the defensive behavior) is in and of itself a hopeful step toward change.

RECOMMENDED MATERIALS FOR GROUP LEADER

Chapter 5 of *Motivational Interviewing* (Miller & Rollnick, 2002) succinctly reviews counselor/client resistance to change relationship patterns. It reviews the same defensive patterns within the context of a professional relationship. This chapter will assist counselors new to the stages of readiness to understand their role in sustaining or moving past clients' dissonant defenses that interfere with the change process.

REQUIRED MATERIALS FOR THE LESSON

- An mp3 player and music selection
- Blackboard, white board, or flip chart
- Markers
- "Common Defenses That Interfere With Knowing How Sexual Life Impacts Recovery" fact sheet (one copy for each participant) (Lesson 2 appendix, A)
- "Sexual Behavior Consciousness Raising Self-Assessment" worksheet (one copy for each participant) (Lesson 2 appendix, B)

OPENING

Opening Music: *Have quiet music playing as participants enter the room and ready themselves (optional).*

Leader: As we sit quietly and focus on being here, let us clear our minds of where we have been and focus on being in this moment.

Opening Poem/Reading:

"Why are you drinking?" demanded the little prince.
"So that I may forget," replied the tippler.
"Forget what?" inquired the little prince, who already was sorry for him.
"Forget that I am ashamed," the tippler confessed, hanging his head.
"Ashamed of what?" insisted the little prince, who wanted to help.
"Ashamed of drinking!" the tippler brought his speech to an end, and shut himself up in an impregnable silence.
And the little prince went away puzzled.
"The grown-ups are certainly very, very odd," he said to himself.

—Antoine De Saint-Exupery, *The Little Prince*

GROUP INTRODUCTION

Have a group member volunteer to read aloud.

Welcome to the sexual health in recovery group. We are here to talk about sex and how our sexual lives affect recovery from drug and alcohol addiction. Some people in recovery risk a relapse because of their sexual behavior at the treatment center or away from the treatment program. This is a place to talk about sexual behavior and sexual health so we can be abstinent from drugs and alcohol. It is also a place to learn about sexual behavior and situations that put men and women in recovery at risk for not completing this treatment program.

Sexual health in recovery is a time to talk about human sexuality and sexual health in a respectful and informed manner. We encourage everyone to be as honest and open as you can be. You are not required to reveal anything about your current or past sexual behavior that would be uncomfortable to discuss. It is important to listen to each other. For some of us, our sexual behavior is the most serious risk to staying in recovery. For others, our sexual behavior gets us into dangerous situations that are triggers to use or drink. A few of us may have little concern about how our sexual behavior contributes to relapse. This group is an opportunity for everyone to learn about the important connection between recovery and sexual health.

LESSON INTRODUCTION

Ask another group member to volunteer to read aloud.

The purpose of today's sexual health in recovery group is to discuss common defense mechanisms that interfere with sexual decisions. Men and women in recovery will increase their likelihood of staying sober when their sexual decisions include honest self-reflection regarding the risk of relapse. Every recovering addict has a responsibility to develop effective sexual decision-making skills as he or she continues maintaining drug and alcohol abstinence in recovery.

Today we will learn skills to overcome barriers for honest self-exploration. Removing these barriers is crucial for assessing our ability to make sexual decisions that reduce the risk of relapse. We will discuss how people in early recovery usually lack the self-awareness to accurately perceive their risks for relapse due to their sexual behavior. We will talk about becoming aware of the defenses used to stay unaware of sex/drug-linked behavior. We will teach you how to identify defenses that interfere with honest self-reflection about sex and drugs. We will role-play how to use the "Sexual Behavior Consciousness Raising Self-Assessment" tool to measure how ready you are to discard your defenses and become aware of your sexual behavior patterns that may lead to relapse.

LECTURE

Leader: How often do you honestly discuss your sexual behavior? How often do you avoid being truthful about your sex life in recovery? Are you interested in learning about how your sexual life will affect your recovery? Do you avoid situations or opportunities to learn more about sexual behavior and recovery? Are you interested in really seeing the consequences, both short-term results and long-term results, of your sexual behavior?

The goal of this group is to normalize resistance to change and to give you some suggestions on how to move beyond defensiveness to look more truthfully at your sexual lives. It isn't easy. Just because we have chosen to enter into a drug and alcohol recovery program does not mean we are equally ready or motivated to look at our sexual selves. In other words, most of us in the room are pretty clear about wanting to address our addiction to drugs and alcohol and begin a program of recovery. We may have been unprepared or unaware of the need to discuss our sexual lives.

Many of you have probably heard or have been told a variety of messages about sex, relationships, falling in love, masturbation, and sexual satisfaction in early recovery. Let's brainstorm a list of things the recovery community has taught you to think when it comes to having sex in sobriety.

Leader asks group for suggestions and writes the list on the board. Examples may be:

- *Sponsor says no sex in first year of sobriety.*
- *Don't have a new relationship the first year of sobriety.*
- *Sex will not be the same as when you were high.*
- *Sex will be a disappointment because you're not high.*
- *You will feel too embarrassed to have the kind of sex you want to have unless you are high or drunk.*
- *It doesn't matter what you do sexually; just don't use.*
- *Masturbate as often as you want if you need to have sex.*
- *Sex can take you out, so be careful.*
- *Watch out for the so-called Thirteen Steppers. Note: "Thirteenth-stepping" is a euphemistic term used among members of Alcoholics Anonymous (AA) to refer to people (particularly men) who target new, more vulnerable members (typically women) for dates or sex (Bogart & Pearce, 2003, p. 43). The term is not gender nor sexual orientation specific within sexual health in recovery. Exploitive sex is a significant boundary-crossing pattern among people in recovery not limited to members of AA.*

Leader: What do you think when look at this list? Are you aware of any thoughts or reactions that go through your mind?

Invite participants to share their thoughts. Have a brief discussion.

Leader: I am going to offer some possible reactions people may have when they hear these common messages about sex or relationships in early recovery.

- I think this is way overblown; not everyone is going to relapse because they have a relationship.
- Sometimes I am really horny and I am going to want to have sex with someone.
- Some people flirt all the time and are so aggressive I just give in so they stop pestering me to have sex with them.

- My sexual life is fine; it really has nothing to do with my addiction
- You are just paranoid and have some serious sexual hang-ups; stop laying your hang-ups on me.
- I am married, so this does not apply to me.
- I am married, so am I supposed to have sex or not? What do I do?

People who are not really ready to discuss their sexual behavior usually react defensively when the subject comes up. Reacting defensively is when we either consciously or unconsciously use behaviors, thoughts, feelings, perceptions, or attitudes to prevent ourselves from knowing something about ourselves. These defenses interfere with our ability to change behavior. If we remain unaware of our defenses, especially the defenses we most frequently rely on, our risk for relapse will increase. What are some defenses you have observed in yourself or people around you when the subject of sex comes up?

Have a brief discussion of examples that participants offer. These may include:

- *Stating an opinion about what is recovery and what is not recovery when it comes to the first year of sobriety and sexuality. It is common to have very strong opinions about sexuality in the first year of recovery. Opinions combined with shaming comments, such as "You shouldn't be focused on that; you need to get sober," may be common responses from counselors and clients.*
- *Making jokes, sexual innuendo, seductive comments, overly familiar sexual humor, or flirtatious behavior can also be common defenses. Creating a sexualized conversation may be an attempt to distract from sex/drug-linked relapse risk. Participants may have many stories about counselors, 12-step fellowship members, sponsors, or friends joking about a history of sex on drugs and minimizing the worry of this link by trivializing the seriousness of the conversation.*
- *Maintaining a tone in the treatment environment that talking about sexual concerns is nothing more than gossip. Participants may have experienced sexual discussion among the other clients as primarily focused on who is attracted to whom, crushes, infatuations, or who may be secretly dating. Leader responses should focus on identifying the defense rather than focusing on the specific content. This discussion is a time to experience observing defenses, not to address the situations or concerns connected to the defensive behavior.*

EXPERIENTIAL LEARNING

Leader: Now let's look at a list of the most common defenses or behaviors experts on addiction have identified.

Hand out the "Common Defenses That Interfere With Knowing How Sexual Life Impacts Recovery" information sheet (Lesson 2 appendix, A). Write the list on board as well.

Leader: We will start at the top of the list and ask for examples of each defense and how it may sound if someone was using this defense when talking about his or her sexual life as it relates to recovery.

The first defense on the list is minimizing. As the worksheet says, this is when someone acknowledges some level of concern about sexual life but discounts this concern as not very significant or very serious. What sort of comments have you heard people make about their sexual lives that acknowledge some concern about their sobriety but make sure that you think the concern is overblown? What have they said? Think about what aspect of their sexual lives they are afraid to discuss in relation to risk for relapse.

Take examples from participants and ask them to highlight the concern that is being minimized as it relates to recovery.

Go through all the other defenses on the list and have two examples of each defense as it relates to sex and recovery given by the participants. For each example, have the participants see if they can highlight the part of the example that describes the defense they are talking about.

Leader: Now that we have gone through each of these defenses, let's talk about how you can put this information to work. Experts who study the process of change find that curiosity and interest in information and stories from people who have made the change that you are thinking about is the best place to start. Being curious and interested in how others have changed is a valuable way to avoid the pitfalls of our defensive responses that prevent moving toward change. Behaviors that help us contemplate if a sexual behavior may put us at risk for relapse include:

(Write this list on the board or have a prepared list that you can post.)

■ Look for information related to sexual behavior in recovery.

- Understand the sexual behavior guidelines for my treatment program.
- Think about the information from the sexual health in recovery program.
- Practice a recovery tool from the sexual health in recovery program.
- Talk with people who have successfully changed their sexual behavior and reduced their risk for relapse.
- Look for information related to sexual behavior in recovery.
- Use tools to understand my defenses that prevent me from changing.

Leader: Just like any behavior, the more we practice the better we become at the behavior. So the more frequently you use the tools listed here, the more likely you will become less defensive and make more informed decisions about your sexual behavior in recovery.

I am now going to hand out a tool you can use to help you measure the frequency that you use consciousness raising about sex and recovery. This worksheet is like a checkpoint for information about yourself to self-correct behavior that is delaying your progress toward making change. The lower your score, the more likely you are remaining pretty unaware of the role sexual behavior can play in early recovery. Not knowing this information can make holding onto your defensive behavior a lot easier. Remember our defenses are needed so we remain unaware of ourselves. Being unaware of our sexual selves is a significant risk for addicts who want to stay clean and sober.

Hand out the "Sexual Behavior Consciousness Raising Self Assessment" form (Lesson 2 appendix, B). Read through the instructions aloud.

TOPIC SKILL PRACTICE

Leader: Now let's do a brief role-play to practice using the "Sexual Behavior Consciousness Raising Self-Assessment" worksheet. I need a volunteer who wants to practice filling out this sheet.

Have a volunteer come to the front of the class.

Leader: I will ask you each a question. I want you to answer each question by rating the frequency of your behavior in the past week.

I will ask you to describe how you rated yourself by giving examples of the behavior. After we go through all four items, we will score your frequency.

> *Ask each question on the worksheet and allow the volunteer to offer an answer. For any item that was answered "never" or "seldom," ask the volunteer to look over the defensive behaviors description checklist and see if she can identify a defense she may use that accounts for the behavior not being more frequent. For example, if the volunteer said she never talks with anyone who has successfully changed her sexual behavior to stay sober, see if she identifies with denial, minimization, or rationalizing as a defense she may use.*
>
> *Invite discussion from other participants about the defenses they may use that might keep their use of the tools for changing sexual relapse prevention behavior at a low frequency.*

Leader: OK, now let's each take a few moments to fill out the "Sexual Behavior Consciousness Raising Self-Assessment" worksheet.

> *Have participants fill out the form and score their answers. For participants who score less than 13, ask them to consider one defense on the defense sheets they think keeps them from scoring higher. For participants who score over 13, ask them to consider one defense that they think they could use less often to get a higher score. Example: Perhaps someone scores 8, and they thought the defense they used a lot was hostility. The group member may discuss ways to reduce using hostility when someone wants to give feedback about their sexual behavior patterns. If someone scores 14, and he or she thought the defense he or she often uses was blaming something outside of him or her, he or she may make a goal to ask others how they reduced using blaming as a defense.*

Leader: You can use this worksheet at anytime to measure your frequency of consciousness raising regarding sexual behavior and relapse risk. If you are concerned about your ability to be really honest with yourself when filling this out, make an appointment with your counselor and you can fill it out together. Remember that the more aware you are about your defenses and the more interested you are in how people in recovery avoid relapse due to sexual behavior or relationships, the more ready you will be to understand your own relapse prevention behavior.

CLOSING

Leader: Now let's take a moment to bring the workshop to a close. Let's take a moment to again quiet ourselves, take a deep breath to quiet our minds, our hearts, and our spirits. In this quiet place, remind yourself how valuable it is to take the time to be honest, vulnerable, and committed to recovery. As you leave the group today, remind yourself that a satisfying sexual life is a vital and important part of recovery. The self-reflection and tools you learned today may become an important part of maintaining your recovery.

REFERENCES

Anderson, D. J. (1981). *The psychopathology of denial*. Minneapolis, MN: Hazeldon.

Bogart, C., & Pearce, C. (2003). "13th-Stepping": Why alcoholics anonymous is not always a safe place for women. *Journal of Addictions Nursing, 14*(1), 43–47.

de Saint-Exupery, A. (1943). *The little prince* (Trans. K. Woods). New York: Reynal & Hitchcock.

Miller, W., & Rollnick, S. (2002). *Motivational interviewing: Preparing people for change* (2nd ed.). New York: The Guilford Press.

Prochaska, J., Norcross, J., & DiClemente, C. (1994). *Changing for good: A revolutionary six-stage program for overcoming bad habits and moving your life positively forward*. New York: Avon Books.

LESSON 2 APPENDIX

A. Common Defenses That Interfere With Knowing How Sexual Life Impacts Recovery

Minimizing: Acknowledge some level of concern about sexual life but discount this concern as not very significant or very serious.

Rationalizing: Present plausible explanations to justify, excuse, or explain sexual behavior.

Intellectualizing: Avoid painful feelings and emotional reactions, and make the sexual situation less personal by using unemotional intellectual analysis.

Blaming: Focus on events outside of one's self and focus on other people, events, or circumstances as a cause or responsibility for sexual behavior or decisions. Personal responsibility for sexual actions and choices is rejected.

Your Basic Everyday Run-of-the-Mill Denial: Insist that one's sexual decision making is not a significant concern for recovery despite a significant amount of evidence that disputes this conclusion. An ongoing effort to filter out information that might make a person consider changing his or her sexual behavior.

Hostility: Become irritated, mean, critical, angry, sullen, temperamental, or shaming toward anyone who invites you to look at your sexual behavior. The purpose for these reactions is to discourage the person from ever bringing up the subject again.

Diversion: Create a flurry of concern about other issues (like whether or not someone loves you or is attracted to you) to make sure there isn't time or ability to focus on one's sexual behavior and the effect it has on recovery. (Adapted from Anderson, 1981, pp. 11–12)

B. Sexual Behavior Consciousness Raising Self-Assessment

This is a brief self-assessment checklist. Each item is a description of a behavior. Rate yourself on the frequency that you have engaged in the behavior in the last 7 days. Choose the number that most closely reflects how frequently you have used this method of sexual behavior consciousness raising. The level of frequency of using these consciousness raising behaviors is a reflection of how ready you are to honestly evaluate your sexual choices and their effect on your sobriety.

1 = Never; 2 = Seldom; 3 = Occasionally; 4 = Often; 5 = Repeatedly

_____I look for information related to sexual behavior in recovery and understand the sexual behavior guidelines for my treatment program.

_____I think about the information from sexual health in recovery and used one of the recovery tools.

_____I talk to people who have successfully changed their sexual behavior and reduced their risk for relapse.

_____I recall information from the sexual health in recovery class and what other people in the class have said about the benefits of changing their sexual behavior.

The highest score is 20.

The higher your score, the more ready you may be to look at your sex/drug-linked relapse risk. Generally people who are not interested in how their sexual behavior may place them at risk for relapse have defenses that interfere with honest self-reflection.

If your scored less than 13, it is recommended that you spend more time increasing your awareness and consciousness about your sexual behavior as a factor in maintaining your recovery.

If you scored more than 13, write down an activity you can focus on over the next week to increase the frequency of your consciousness raising behavior.

_____

_____

_____

_____

_____

(Adapted from Prochaska et al., 1994, p. 93)

3

Dating and Sexual Relationships in Recovery

CORE CONCEPT

Women and men in recovery routinely worry about their current or future relationships with partners or spouses. What does a relationship in recovery look like? Whether you are currently in a relationship, married, dating, single, or widowed, women and men in recovery increase their likelihood of staying sober when they prepare for sexual health skills in dating and relationships. Today's class will start by looking back on our history with dating, falling in love, and our use of drugs and alcohol. The remainder of the class will be divided into two groups. One group will be single, dating, divorced, or widowed group members. The second group will be men and women currently in a long-term partnership or marriage. Each group will learn 10 common myths about relationships and dating in recovery. You will learn a key sexual health question and key sexual health recovery tool to address each myth. Each group will practice the "Ready for Dating and Recovery Worksheet" (Lesson 3 appendix, A) or the "Recovery in Marriage or Relationship Worksheet" (Lesson 3 appendix, B).

BELIEF STATEMENT

Sexual health in recovery is the ability to prepare for sexual health skills in dating and relationships.

OBJECTIVES

Participants will
- Divide into coupled and single groups.
- Discuss myths about relationships and dating in recovery.
- Learn the 10 key sexual health questions about relationships and dating in recovery.
- Learn to use the "Ready for Dating and Recovery Worksheet" and "Recovery in Marriage or Relationship Worksheet" assessment tools

CHANGE GOALS

- Integrate honest self-reflection regarding risk of relapse into sexual decisions.
- Learn common defense mechanisms that interfere with honest self-reflection.
- Understand common myths about recovery and relationships.

REQUIRED READING FOR GROUP LEADER

- *Awakening Your Sexuality*, by Covington (2000). In Chapter 7 (pp. 119–139) "Understanding Partner Selection," author Stephanie Covington reviews significant relationship and dating in recovery themes. The chapter provides the group leader with recovery-focused issues for women looking honestly at their current or ideal future relationship. Covington reinforces several key concepts in the myths about dating and relationships that will support the group leader in addressing the central message that becoming clean and sober does not lead directly to changes in relationships, marriages, or dating patterns.

■ *The Seven Principles of Making Marriage Work,* by Gottman and Silver (1999), is a source for research-based fundamental relationship skills. A portion of this book is adapted for Lesson 12 (Body Image). I recommend reading chapters 1 and 2, which focus on both ends of the relationship spectrum. In the first chapter the authors describe their research observations about constructive and deadly relationship patterns. The second chapter is useful for the group leader to have specific relationship pattern information that is highly correlated with eroding relationships and that almost always lead to divorce. In early recovery men and women benefit from specific, factual, and basic information to sustain relationships.

RECOMMENDED MATERIALS FOR GROUP LEADER

■ *A General Theory of Love,* by Lewis, Amini, and Lannon (2001), is a book that transformed the way I think about love. The authors set out to answer questions about love found within the hearts deepest vessels, hidden and waiting to be known. Elegantly interweaving literature, brain science, attachment theory, and neural learning these scientist-poets-of-love invite us to ponder: "Who we are and who we become depends, in part, on whom we love" (p. 144). I find their invitation to understand the process of emotional healing through relationship enormously reflective of the basic beliefs of recovery and sexual health. They have much science to back up what the recovery community believes. I have never ceased having a limbic connection with this book.

REQUIRED MATERIALS FOR THE LESSON

■ An mp3 player and music selection.
■ Index cards preprinted with the myths of dating in recovery (one set for each participant) (see "Experiential Learning" section for the text to be printed on each card).
■ Index cards preprinted with the myths of marriage and relationships in recovery (one set for each participant) (see "Experiential Learning" section for the text to be printed on each card).
■ "Ready for Dating and Recovery Worksheet" (one copy for each participant) (Lesson 3 appendix, A).

- "Recovery in Marriage or Relationship Worksheet" (one copy for each participant) (Lesson 3 appendix, B).
- "Stop, Think, Inform, Listen, and Listen (STILL)" recovery tool (one copy for each participant) (Lesson 3 appendix, C).

OPENING

Opening Music: *Have quiet music playing as participants enter the room and ready themselves (optional).*

Leader: As we sit quietly and focus on being here, let us clear our minds of where we have been and focus on being in this moment.

Opening Poem/Reading:

I love you,
Not only for what you are,
But for what I am when I am with you.
I love you,
Not only for what you have made of yourself,
But for what you are making of me.
I love you for the part of me that you bring out;
I love you for putting your hand into my heaped-up heart and passing over all the foolish, weak things that you can't help dimly seeing there,
And for drawing out into the light all the beautiful belongings that no one else had looked quite far enough to find.
I love you because you are helping me to make of the lumber of my life not a tavern but a temple;
Out of the works of my every day not a reproach but a song.
I love you because you have done more than any creed could have done to make me good and more than any fate could have done to make me happy.
You have done it without a touch, without a word, without a sign.
You have done it by being yourself.
Perhaps that is what being a friend means, after all.

—Roy Croft, *I Love You*

GROUP INTRODUCTION

Have a group member volunteer to read aloud.

Welcome to the sexual health in recovery group. We are here to talk about sex and how our sexual lives affect recovery from drug and alcohol addiction. Some people in recovery risk a relapse because of their sexual behavior at the treatment center or away from the treatment program. This is a place to talk about sexual behavior and sexual health so we can be abstinent from drugs and alcohol. It is also a place to learn about sexual behavior and situations that put men and women in recovery at risk for not completing this treatment program.

Sexual health in recovery is a time to talk about human sexuality and sexual health in a respectful and informed manner. We encourage everyone to be as honest and open as you can be. You are not required to reveal anything about your current or past sexual behavior that would be uncomfortable to discuss. It is important to listen to each other. For some of us, our sexual behavior is the most serious risk to staying in recovery. For others, our sexual behavior gets us into dangerous situations that are triggers to use or drink. A few of us may have little concern about how our sexual behavior contributes to relapse. This group is an opportunity for everyone to learn about the important connection between recovery and sexual health.

LESSON INTRODUCTION

Ask another group member to volunteer to read aloud.

The purpose of today's sexual health in recovery group is to discuss relationships in recovery. Women and men in early recovery often experience worries and fears about their current relationship with their partner or spouse. Single men and women may experience similar fears and concerns about meeting, dating, or falling in love in recovery. Everyone in recovery must eventually face either rebuilding a current relationship, building a new found love, or accepting their limitations and capacity for love and connection. Men and women in recovery will increase their likelihood of staying sober when they learn sexual health skills in dating and relationships. Whether married, domestic partnered, single, divorced, separated, widowed, dating, or just completely not interested in romance, relationship skills are central to the process of recovery. We will begin by looking back on our history with dating. We will focus on our drug and alcohol use during dating. The class will then divide into two groups. Single, dating, divorced, or widowed women and men will be in one group. The other group will be men and women currently married, registered domestic partners, or in a long-term relationship.

It is a myth that staying sober and beginning the recovery process will automatically result in dating and relationship skills. Sexual health in recovery includes looking at sex/drug-linked relationship patterns in our addiction and understanding the risk for relapse if these patterns are not changed. Each group will learn 10 myths about relationships and dating in recovery. We will learn to ask important sexual health questions and to utilize a key relationship sexual health tool for each sexual health question. Each group will practice the "Ready for Dating and Recovery Worksheet" or the "Recovery in Marriage or Relationship Worksheet" as sexual health tools for finding and staying in love.

LECTURE (WITH ENTIRE GROUP)

Leader: Whether you are currently in a relationship, married, dating, single, or widowed, we will start today by looking back on our history with dating, falling in love, and our use of drugs and alcohol. What is a date? Dating is when a pair or even a group socialize and interact with the aim of each person evaluating the other as a possible person with whom to fall in love or as a potential spouse. What is the best date you ever had? Think for a moment, remember the date and focus on what made it so wonderful.

Lead a discussion with the group on the wonderful elements of a date. Were drugs or alcohol involved? What was the worst date you ever had? What made it so bad? Were drugs or alcohol involved?

Leader: We have all had some experience with dating, some with being in relationships and, others may currently be in a relationship or marriage. For the remainder of the class, we will divide into two groups that will meet in separate rooms. Those who consider themselves currently single, dating, divorced, or widowed are one group. Those who are currently in a relationship or legally married will be in the other group.

Have the participants split up into two groups. Each group will be led by at least one facilitator. Each group has a separate curriculum for the remainder of the lesson.

EXPERIENTIAL LEARNING (SINGLE, DATING, DIVORCED, WIDOWED GROUP)

Leader: We will start our small group discussion by introducing myths about dating in recovery.

Hand out the myths of dating in recovery cards, which should be prepared prior to the lesson. On one side of each card is a myth. On the other side will be facts that refute the myth, as well as a key sexual health question and a key sexual health in recovery tool.

Have a group member draw a card and read the myth out loud. Lead a group discussion on the myth. Base discussion on the facts listed on the back of the card. Guide the group to keep discussion focused on their current situations with dating and recovery. Watch for the defense of intellectualizing (talking about the idea without personal self-disclosure or discussion). Limit discussion with each myth to no more than 10 minutes. Groups should complete a minimum of five myths. A second session can be scheduled to complete discussion of all 10 myths.

Here are suggested responses and discussion points for each of the dating in recovery myths:

Myth 1: Being in recovery and staying sober will change the type of person I am attracted to
Facts

- Being in recovery will first and foremost help you treat your addiction and lead a sober life.
- Drug and alcohol recovery is a lifelong process of recovery. Our attractions, whom we imagine falling or being in love with, are imprinted in our minds and souls from influential relationships when we were quite young.
- Being sober will help us discover who we are but will not be a formula for changing these imprinted relationship maps deep in our psyche that determine when or with whom we feel attraction.
- Key sexual health question: Do I know that my early life history will affect my attractions and love fantasies?
- Key sexual health in recovery tool: Talk about my dating and relationship history with a minimum of three people in my recovery support system.

Myth 2: Being in recovery will give me a clear picture of how to recognize an unhealthy attraction
Facts

- Being in recovery will first and foremost help you treat your addiction and lead a sober life.
- This is the first and foremost concern for a single, divorced, or widowed person in recovery: Will I only be attracted to someone

who is using or drinking? Will attractions to someone using or drinking put my sobriety at risk?
- Focusing on when I feel attractions to someone who is not high or drinking is the recovery tool. It may be surprising to experience feeling attraction to someone who is sober.
- Key sexual health question: Do I have patterns in my attractions that are a threat or risk for sobriety?
- Key sexual health in recovery tool: Noticing feelings of attraction when in sober situations where no one is drinking or high.

Myth 3: Being in recovery will keep me open-minded and ready for feedback from others about my unhealthy attraction
Facts
- Being in recovery is a crash course in a lifelong skill of treating addiction. Being open-minded about and ready for feedback about what may risk sobriety is hard enough.
- Being open and willing to go to any lengths to stay sober may not always include being open to feedback about your dating patterns and behavior.
- Key sexual health question: Do I get defensive and mistrustful when my support system gives me feedback about my risk for relapse and thinking about dating or going on a date?
- Key sexual health in recovery tool: Listen to feedback from my recovery support system about my defensive reactions when discussing my attractions and plans to date. Use the "Common Defenses That Interfere With Knowing How Sexual Life Impacts Recovery" sheet (from Lesson 2).

Myth 4: Being in recovery will protect me from having unmanageable emotional attractions
Facts
- Recovery is a process of learning how to have intense emotional feelings and manage these feelings without resorting to using drugs and alcohol.
- Anyone who is committed to sobriety and recovery is going to have a wide variety of feelings that may at the time seem unmanageable.
- Feeling of attractions, desire, having a crush, lusting for someone, loving someone, and dreams about someone are all part of life and part of recovery.

- What protects a person in recovery from having unmanageable feelings is talking about them in a safe and nonshaming place or relationship.
- Key sexual health question: Do I have a support circle that I can trust to discuss my intense feelings of attraction?
- Key sexual health in recovery tool: Use my support circle to complete the "Stop, Think, Inform, Listen, and Listen (STILL)" recovery tool.

Myth 5: Being in recovery will give me the proper guidelines for selecting a good relationship
Facts

- If there was such a thing as the proper guidelines for selecting someone to date, everyone would follow them. Or would they?
- The problem with thinking there is a right way to go about dating is that it does not put the focus on you!
- As we will see in our recovery skills for dating, focusing on yourself and developing who you are as a person is a much more important focus.
- Key sexual health question: Would I want to date me?
- Key sexual health in recovery tool: Know signs of behavior and attitudes of the people I date that are serious signs of not supporting my recovery.

Myth 6: If you are single, staying clean and sober for a year before doing any dating is the best approach to love and sexual relationships in recovery
Facts

- This magical boundary is the source of much power struggles, secrecy, shame, and conflict with sponsors.
- We do know that when a person stays clean and sober for 1 year, it greatly increases his or her chances of remaining committed to a lifelong program of recovery.
- We know that dating and forming relationships without a clear plan for staying sober is a serious risk for recovery. The recovery community and drug and alcohol treatment field has perpetuated the ideal of 365 days without dating or sexual activity as an unquestioned recovery tool.
- There is nothing magical about a year of being clean and sober to be ready for relationships. Knowing your dating in sobriety personal relapse risk factors is a much more important skill.

- Key sexual health question: Do I know what I may need to change in myself to be ready for dating and staying sober?
- Key recovery tool: Complete all the tasks of the "Ready for Dating and Recovery Worksheet."

Myth 7: I can learn what I need to know about dating from books, sponsors, and friends
Facts

- We can learn what self-help books suggest, we can learn what worked for our sponsor, we can learn from our friends' experiences, but it may not be what *we* need to learn.
- This class will focus on a three-step process for evaluating your readiness for dating and staying sober.
- We learned our most ingrained relationship patterns *in* relationships; we will learn new and different patterns *in* relationships as well.
- Key sexual health question: Do I know how to evaluate my readiness for dating and staying sober?
- Key sexual health in recovery tool: Share your completed "Ready for Dating and Recovery Worksheet" with at least two helpers.

Myth 8: I can learn what I need to know about dating fairly quickly without making the same blunders over and over again
Facts

- "Can somebody survey a group and intuit who has a bad temper, an alcoholic mother, who dreams at night of revenge on the father who left him? Look at the relationships around you and judge for yourself. People target the mates who mesh with their own minds" (Lewis et al., 2001, p. 161).
- If we really want to learn about dating we have to go through the process of struggle and mess that comes from placing ourselves in dating situations where we will feel all the emotions and thoughts that happen when we make an effort to emotionally connect with someone with whom we feel attracted.
- Key sexual health question: Do I have the recovery tools I need to deal with the emotions and thoughts I will have when dating?
- Key sexual health in recovery tool: Continue using the "Ready for Dating and Recovery Worksheet" to focus on the patterns of behavior and attitudes you continue to repeat that place your sobriety at risk.

Myth 9: Dating too early in recovery is a dangerous relapse risk
Facts

- Dating is not the risk; being unprepared for relapse triggers without an adequate support system in the risk.
- Inadequate sexual health recovery tools are a significant reason many people have difficulty with being sober and dating.
- Just like anything in sobriety, being prepared for relapse triggers is the key to staying sober.
- This class will give you the "Ready for Dating and Recovery Worksheet" assessment tool as a practical resource you can use over and over again to assess your preparation for dating this person, at this time, and at this point in your sobriety.
- Key sexual health question: Am I interested in using the "Ready for Dating and Recovery Worksheet"?
- Key sexual health in recovery tool: The "Ready for Dating and Recovery Worksheet."

Myth 10: Being in recovery is a good short cut for learning dating and sexual relationship skills
Facts

- Being in recovery is not really a short cut to anything.
- Being in recovery is hard work and a serious commitment to your health and well-being.
- The longer you are in recovery, the more you know that there are no short cuts for staying sober.
- The longer you stay in recovery, the more you know about recovery. Recovery skills improve with practice.
- The same is true about dating. It takes a serious commitment to maintain your health and well-being and dive into the emotional sea of attractions, sexuality, and love.
- Millions of people are in recovery. Millions of people date, fall in love, and form relationships. Putting this into perspective can help.
- Key sexual health question: Am I prepared and ready to do the time-consuming and slow work of learning how to combine sexually healthy dating into my recovery?
- Key sexual health in recovery tool: Completing the "Ready for Dating and Recovery Worksheet" as many times as needed before acting on an attraction.

Complete at least five dating in recovery myth cards before transitioning the group to the "Ready for Dating and Recovery Worksheet." The remainder of the group will focus on teaching how to use and fill out this recovery tool.

TOPIC SKILL PRACTICE

Hand out the "Ready for Dating and Recovery" Worksheet (Lesson 3 appendix, A).

Leader: This worksheet can be completed as an inventory of your current readiness to begin dating in recovery. Look at each item and examine readiness to do this particular sexual health in recovery tool. Check the box that best describes your readiness to complete this sexual health relapse prevention skill. The more tools you have completed, the more ready you are to consider dating in recovery without a serious relapse risk.

Lead group discussion before closing workshop. Focus discussion on items group members have checked as "done" or "getting ready." Have group members discuss what tasks or actions need to be completed so that a "getting ready" item can move to "done." Have members focus on which of the 10 tasks is the most crucial for each group member to avoid relapse.

CLOSING

Leader: Now let's take a moment to bring the workshop to a close. Let's take a moment to again quiet ourselves, take a deep breath to quiet our minds, our hearts, and our spirits. In this quiet place, remind yourself how valuable it is to take the time to be honest, vulnerable, and committed to recovery. As you leave the group today, remind yourself that a satisfying sexual life is a vital and important part of recovery. The self-reflection and tools you learned today may become an important part of maintaining your recovery.

EXPERIENTIAL LEARNING (MARRIED OR RELATIONSHIP GROUP)

Leader: We will start our small group discussion by introducing myths about marriage and relationships in recovery.

Hand out the myths of marriage and relationships in recovery cards, which should be prepared prior to the lesson. On one side of each card is a myth. On the other side will be the facts that refute the myth, as well as a key sexual health question and a key sexual health in recovery tool.

Have a group member draw a card and read the myth out loud. Lead a group discussion on the myth. Base discussion on the facts listed on the back of the card. Guide the group to keep discussion focused on their current situations with relationships and recovery. Watch for the defense of intellectualizing (talking about the idea without personal self-disclosure or discussion). Limit discussion with each myth to no more than 10 minutes. Groups should complete a minimum of five myths. A second session can be scheduled to complete discussion of all 10 myths.

Here are suggested responses and discussion points for each of the myths:

Myth 1: Being in recovery and staying sober will change the type of partner I am in my relationship or marriage
Facts

- Being in recovery will first and foremost help you treat your addiction and lead a sober life.
- Drug and alcohol recovery is a lifelong process of recovery. Who we are in a relationship and the history of our current marriage has left a mark and will take time to understand.
- Being sober will help us discover who we are but will not be a formula for changing these relationship maps that are deep in our psyches.
- Key sexual health question: Do I know that my early life history will affect my attractions and love fantasies in my current relationship?
- Key sexual health recovery tool: Talk about my dating and relationship history of my current and past relationships with a minimum of three people in my recovery support system.

Myth 2: Being in recovery will give me a clear picture of how to recognize an unhealthy relationship or marriage
Facts

- Being in recovery will first and foremost help you treat your addiction and lead a sober life.
- This is the first and foremost concern for a married or coupled woman or man in recovery: Is my relationship too unhealthy to stay sober?

- Focusing on the link between my marriage or relationship and my sobriety is a much more useful question.
- Key sexual health question: Do I have behavior patterns in my marriage or relationship that are a threat or risk for sobriety?
- Key sexual health in recovery tool: Using the "Stopping and Thinking About Sex/Drug Situations in Recovery Worksheet" (from Lesson 1).

Myth 3: Being in recovery will keep me open-minded and ready for feedback from others about my unhealthy attractions for someone other than my current partner or spouse
Facts

- Being in recovery is a crash course in a lifelong skill of treating addiction. Being open-minded about and ready for feedback about what may risk sobriety is hard enough.
- Being open and willing to go to any lengths to stay sober may not always include being ready or open to feedback about your relationship or marriage patterns and behavior.
- Key sexual health question: Do I get defensive and mistrustful when my support system gives me feedback about my risk for relapse due to patterns and behavior in my relationship or marriage?
- Key sexual health recovery tool: Listen to feedback from my recovery support system about my defensive reactions when discussing my behavior in my relationship or marriage.

Myth 4: Being in recovery will protect me from having unmanageable emotional attractions for someone other than my current partner or spouse
Facts

- Recovery is a process of learning how to have intense emotional feelings and manage these feelings without resorting to using drugs and alcohol.
- Anyone who is committed to sobriety and recovery is going to have a wide variety of feelings that may at the time seem unmanageable.
- Feeling of attractions, desire, having a crush, lusting for someone, or having love dreams for someone other than my current partner or spouse are all part of life and part of recovery.
- What protects a person in recovery from destructive behavior in coping with unmanageable feelings is talking about them in a safe and nonshaming place or relationship.

- Key sexual health question: Do I have a support circle that I can trust to discuss my intense sexual feelings?
- Key sexual health recovery tool: Use my support circle to complete the "Stop, Think, Inform, Listen, and Listen (STILL)" recovery tool

Myth 5: Being in recovery will give me the proper guidelines for maintaining a good relationship or a good marriage
Facts

- If all it took to maintain a good marriage was following the proper guidelines for maintaining a good marriage or relationship, everyone would follow them. Or would they?
- The problem with thinking there is a right way to go about a long-term relationship or marriage is that it does not put the focus on you!
- As we will see in our recovery skills for relationship and marriage, focusing on yourself and developing who you are as a person is a much more important focus.
- Key sexual health question: Would I want to be in a relationship or marriage with me?
- Key sexual health recovery tool: Develop four or five basic relationship skills for maintaining your recovery.

Myth 6: If you are currently coupled or married, staying clean and sober 12 months before making any significant decisions about your current marriage or relationship is the best approach
Facts

- This magical boundary of 1 year is the source of much debate, secrecy, shame, and conflict with sponsors.
- We do know that when a person stays clean and sober for 1 year, it greatly increases his or her chances of remaining committed to a lifelong program of recovery.
- We know that men and women currently coupled or married without a clear plan for staying sober have a serious risk for staying sober.
- There is nothing magical about a year of being clean and sober to be ready to make significant changes in a relationship.
- A newly sober person's recovery may be at risk because of serious and dangerous relationship circumstances. Items that must

be addressed early in recovery include: Violence in the couple, partner use of drugs, alcohol, untreated severe mental illness, untreated drug and alcohol dependency, compulsive gambling, out-of-control sexual behavior, illegal and criminal behavior, sexual abuse of children, sexual activity with minors, history of rape or forced sex in the relationship, threats of harm to children, forced termination of pregnancy, undisclosed sexually transmitted infection, sexual behavior putting partner at risk for HIV infection, deceptive use or discontinuance of contraception, affairs, and sexual activity that violated the boundaries of the primary relationship. Any one of these circumstances left unaddressed poses a significant risk to sobriety. If left unaddressed early in recovery or delayed, ignored, denied, or purposely hidden, it will doom sobriety. Knowing what relationship or marriage stressors are personal relapse risk factors and the direct impact they do and will have on your sobriety is a much more important skill than rigidly adhering to no action until 12 months after sobriety.

- Key sexual health question: Do I know what I may need to change in myself to be ready to face painful, difficult, and sobriety-threatening circumstances and secrets in my relationship or marriage?
- Key sexual health recovery tool: Complete all the tasks of the "Recovery in Marriage or Relationship" inventory.

Myth 7: I can learn what I need to know about being a recovering couple or marriage from books, sponsors, and friends
Facts

- We can learn what self-help books suggest, we can learn what worked for our sponsor, we can learn from our friends' experiences, but it may not be what *you* need to learn.
- We learned our most ingrained relationship patterns *in* relationships; we will learn new and different patterns *in* relationships as well.
- Key sexual health question: Do I know how to evaluate my relationship or marital patterns that will enhance sexual health and maintain recovery?
- Key sexual health recovery tool: Complete all the tasks for the "Ready for Recovery in Marriage or Relationship Worksheet" inventory.

Myth 8: I can learn what I need to know about sexual health in relationships and marriage fairly quickly without making the same blunders over and over again

Facts

■ "Can somebody survey a group and intuit who has a bad temper, an alcoholic mother, who dreams at night of revenge on the father who left him? Look at the relationships around you and judge for yourself. People target the mates who mesh with their own minds" (Lewis et al., 2001, p. 161).

■ When we make an effort to emotionally connect with a spouse or partner after years of addiction, we must have some recovery tools to help us manage the feelings and thoughts that will arise.

■ Key sexual health question: Do I have the sexual health recovery tools I need to deal with the emotions and thoughts (that I usually cope with by using) that I will have in my relationship or marriage?

■ Key sexual health in recovery tool: Utilize my support system to manage intense feelings and reactions toward my spouse or partner.

Myth 9: Addressing relationship or marital concerns early in recovery is too much of a relapse risk

Facts

■ Your relationship or marriage is not the relapse risk; being unprepared for your individual relapse triggers associated with looking honestly at your relationship is the real problem.

■ Avoiding relapse preparation when facing relationship or marital concerns in recovery is the reason many people have difficulty with being sober and being married or coupled.

■ Just like anything in sobriety, being prepared for relapse triggers is the key to staying sober.

■ Key sexual health question: Am I interested in using the "Recovery in Marriage and Relationship Worksheet" assessment tool?

■ Key sexual health in recovery tool: This class will give you the "Recovery in Marriage or Relationship Worksheet" assessment tool as a practical resource you can use over and over again to assess your preparation for addressing relationship issues at this time and at this stage of your sobriety.

Myth 10: Being in recovery is a good short cut for learning marriage and sexual relationship skills

Facts

- Being in recovery is not really a short cut to anything.
- Being in recovery is hard work and a serious commitment to your health and well-being.
- The longer you are in recovery, the more you know there are no short cuts for staying sober.
- The longer you stay in recovery, the more you know about recovery. Recovery skills improve with practice.
- The same is true about sex and relationships. It takes a serious commitment to maintain your sobriety and recovery combined with addressing the emotions connected with attractions, desire, sexuality, and love.
- Millions of people are in recovery. Millions of people feel attractions and desire; millions fall in love; millions form relationships. Millions marry. Putting this into perspective can help.
- Key sexual health question: Am I prepared and ready to do the time-consuming and slow work of learning how to be in a couple in recovery?
- Key sexual health in recovery tool: Completing the "Recovery in Marriage or Relationship Worksheet" as many times as needed before implementing significant changes in my marriage or relationship.

TOPIC SKILL PRACTICE

Hand out the "Recovery in Marriage or Relationship Worksheet" (Lesson 3 appendix, B).

Leader: This worksheet can be completed as an inventory of your current readiness and preparation for recovery in marriage or a relationship. Look at each item and examine your stage of readiness to do this particular sexual health in recovery tool. Check the box that best describes your readiness to complete this sexual health relapse prevention skill. The more tools you have completed, the more ready you are for maintaining your recovery in your marriage or current relationship.

Lead group discussion before closing workshop. Focus discussion on items group members checked as "done" or "getting ready." Have group members discuss what tasks or actions need to be completed so that a "getting ready" item can move to "done." Have members focus on which of the 12 tasks are the most crucial for each group member to avoid relapse.

CLOSING

Leader: Now let's take a moment to bring the workshop to a close. Let's take a moment to again quiet ourselves, take a deep breath to quiet our minds, our hearts, and our spirits. In this quiet place, remind yourself how valuable it is to take the time to be honest, vulnerable, and committed to recovery. As you leave the group today, remind yourself that a satisfying sexual life is a vital and important part of recovery. The self-reflection and tools you learned today may become an important part of maintaining your recovery.

REFERENCES

Covington, S. (2000). *Awakening your sexuality: A guide for recovering women.* Center City, MN: Hazelden.

Croft, R. (2009). *I love you.* Retrieved May 22, 2009, from http://thinkexist.com/quotation/i-love-you-not-only-for-what-you-are-but-for-what/1602010.html

Gottman, J., & Silver, N. (1999). *The seven principles for making marriage work.* New York: Three Rivers Press.

Lewis, T., Amini, F., & Lannon, R. (2001). *A general theory of love.* New York: Vintage Books.

LESSON 3 APPENDIX

A. Ready for Dating and Recovery Worksheet

Table 1

READY FOR DATING AND RECOVERY WORKSHEET

	NOT READY	GETTING READY	DONE
Talk about my dating history with a minimum of three people in my recovery support system.			
Talk about my interest in learning more about dating with a minimum of three people in my recovery support.			
Look for information about dating in recovery from books, magazines, Internet recovery chat rooms, therapist, counselor.			
Talk about dating information I am learning with my recovery support system.			
Use the "Stop, Think, Inform, Listen, and Listen (STILL)" tool when feeling attractions.			
Can identify at least two defensive reactions I tend to have when I talk to my support system about dating or relationships.			
Can identify at least two behaviors or attitudes of a dating partner that would be a serious sign of not supporting my recovery.			
Can identify at least two personal information disclosures I will keep to myself until having three dates.			
Can identify at least two things I do well on dates.			

Table 1

READY FOR DATING AND RECOVERY WORKSHEET (CONTINUED)			
	NOT READY	GETTING READY	DONE
Before dating have at least two people in my support system with whom I can talk honestly and openly about my dating experiences.			
Can identify the two biggest mistakes I could make on the first three dates that could risk my sobriety.			
Can identify the two most important recovery tools for me to use on a date.			

B. Recovery in Marriage or Relationship Worksheet

Table 2

RECOVERY IN MARRIAGE OR RELATIONSHIP WORKSHEET

	NOT READY	GETTING READY	DONE
Talk about my relationship and marital history with a minimum of three people in my recovery support system.			
Talk about my interest in learning more about relationships and marriage in recovery with a minimum of three people in my support system.			
Look for information about relationships and marriage in recovery from books, magazines, Internet recovery chat rooms, therapist, counselor.			
Talk about relationship or marriage information I am learning with my recovery support system.			
Use the "Stop, Think, Listen, and Listen (STILL)" tool when feeling attractions.			
Can identify at least two defensive reactions I tend to have when I talk to my support system about my relationship or marriage.			
Can identify at least two behaviors or attitudes of my partner or spouse that would be a serious sign of not supporting my recovery.			
Can identify at least two personal information disclosures I will keep to myself until I have a relapse prevention plan in place.			
Can identify at least two skills I do well in my relationship or marriage.			

Table 2

RECOVERY IN MARRIAGE OR RELATIONSHIP WORKSHEET (CONTINUED)

	NOT READY	GETTING READY	DONE
Before addressing a significant relationship or marital issue, have at least two support people with whom I can talk honestly and openly.			
Can identify the two biggest mistakes I could make when addressing a relationship or marital concern that could risk my sobriety.			
Can identify the two most important recovery tools for me to use in my relationship or marriage.			

C. Stop, Think, Inform, Listen, and Listen (STILL) Sexual Health in Recovery Worksheet

Acting impulsively without thinking is a common pattern of behavior for men and women in early recovery. STILL is designed to delay impulsive actions in a relationship. Sexual health in recovery is the ability to slow down sexual feelings or attractions to consider the sex/drug link. Taking the time to consider the sex/drug link of a particular sexual situation is central to sexual health in recovery. STILL can be practiced over and over again. STILL is a relationship skill that can be used at any time in recovery.

There are five steps in STILL.

1. Stop
2. Think
3. Inform
4. Listen
5. Listen

Without the first step nothing else can happen. Stop!

Knowing when to stop, take a break, or slow down is a very important tool. Only you can decide to take this step. You have to be the one to decide to stop and notice that a sexual feeling, fantasy, impulse, or plan may need to be evaluated in regard to the link with drugs/alcohol. Sexual health in recovery is taking the time to do this evaluation before taking action.

This worksheet is a guide for what to do after you stop an impulse or urge before taking action.

Think: The thinking step involves answering four questions.

1. What sexual behavior/situation am I thinking about?
2. What aspect of this sexual behavior/situation is high risk for drug/alcohol relapse?
3. What aspect of this sexual behavior/situation is low risk for drug/alcohol relapse?
4. Who in my key support circle do I want to ask to listen to me about this sexual behavior/situation?

When you can answer these four questions go to the next step:

Inform: Take your answers and inform a key trusted member of your support system. This cannot be the person with whom you are having the sexual feelings or interest. Inform your key support person of your situation and answers to the four questions.

Listen: Have him or her listen to your answers to all four questions. The job of your support person is to first listen to your responses. He or she should listen without interruption and should concentrate on hearing your thoughts and assessment of the situation. This is the part where you are listened to.

Listen: The last step is to listen to what your key support person says after listening to you. This is your time to listen without interruption. The key to this skill is to listen. Listening does not mean agreement. Listening does not mean complying. Listening is a form of concentration with the focus on paying attention to what another person is saying. Listening is an effort to hear and take into account what your key support system is saying.

The ability to stop, think, inform, and listen will be a significant skill in improving sexual health in recovery.

Sexual Attitudes and Values

4   Motivations for Sex in Recovery

CORE CONCEPT

New sex research suggests that "motivations for engaging in sexual intercourse may be larger in number and psychologically complex in nature" (Meston & Buss, 2007, p. 477). Men and women in recovery may express reasons for having sex that are similar and different from the general population. Sexual health increases when time is taken for honest reflection about current motivations for sex. Teaching skills for understanding sexual motivations linked with drug/alcohol use is an important recovery tool. Experiential learning incorporating the fun of a Family Feud game format using recent sex research surveys teaches participants to talk about and critically evaluate motivations for sex. The "Stop, Think, Inform, Listen, and Listen (STILL) Sexual Health in Recovery Worksheet" (from Lesson 3) will be utilized as a relapse prevention skill to pause and reflect on motivations for sex in recovery.

BELIEF STATEMENT

Sexual health in recovery is the ability to evaluate level of relapse risk within a wide range of motivations for sex.

OBJECTIVES

Participants will
- Learn new research about motivations for sex.
- Consider how men and women are similar and different in their motivations for sex.
- Identify high-frequency motivations for combining sex and drugs.
- Play a modified version of Family Feud utilizing survey results among workshop participants.
- Complete the "I STILL Want to Have Sex in Recovery Worksheet" using motivations for sex survey information.

CHANGE GOALS

- Normalize differences and similarities between men and women's motivations for sex.
- Utilize sex research to increase knowledge about low- and high-frequency motivations for sex.
- Increase ability to pause and consider sex/drug link when motivated to pursue sex.

REQUIRED READING FOR GROUP LEADER

Meston, C., & Buss, D. (2007). Why humans have sex? *Archives of Sexual Behavior, 36,* 477–507. The motivations for sex as described in this article are the basis for this lesson. If you go to Google and put the title of the article with the question mark you will be able to view the entire article.

RECOMMENDED MATERIALS FOR GROUP LEADER

- "Greater Expectations: Adolescents' Positive Motivations for Sex," by Ott, Millstein, Ofner, & Halpern-Fisher (2006). This lesson is based on adult motivations for sex, however, this article is an excellent overview of sex-positive adolescent motivations for sexual intercourse. The study found that "adolescents view intimacy, sexual pleasure and social status as important goals in a relationship. Many have strong positive expectations that sex would satisfy these goals" (p. 84). For adolescent drug and alcohol treatment programs, this study may be an important resource for adaptation of this lesson. Second, with many addicts beginning a life-long link between sexual activity and drug use in adolescence, this research may assist in discussions that reflect on early sex/drug-linked motivations.

REQUIRED MATERIALS FOR THE LESSON

- An mp3 player and music selection
- 400 unlined colored index cards (100 each green, red, white, and purple), divided into two decks of 200 cards (50 of each color). The colors should not be mixed.
- Clear tape (two rolls)
- Scissors (two pairs)
- Preprinted lists of high-frequency motivations for sex for women and for men (Lesson 4 appendix, A and B), one for each participant
- The "50 Sex/Drug-Linked Motivations for Sexual Intercourse" (Lesson 4 appendix, C), one copy for each participant
- Index cards preprinted with the "Sexual Motivations in Addiction" (see Lesson 4 appendix, C)
- Computer with PowerPoint program and screen projection
- Prepared PowerPoint Family Feud format game (Lesson 4 appendix, D)
- "I STILL Want to Have Sex in Recovery Worksheet" (one copy for each participant) (Lesson 4 appendix, E)

OPENING

Opening Music: *Have quiet music playing as participants enter the room and ready themselves (optional).*

Leader: As we sit quietly and focus on being here, let us clear our minds of where we have been and focus on being in this moment.

Opening Poem/Reading:

Human sexual motivation is an unusual motivation. In lower animals we speak about sexual motivation as a "drive." That is, we state that some internal, innate force pushes the animal to engage in reproductive behavior.

Humans don't simply give in to an internal push towards sexual behavior. Instead, human motivation to engage in sexual behavior is due to a complex relationship among several factors.

—K. Johnson, *Human Sexual Motivation* (1997)

GROUP INTRODUCTION

Have a group member volunteer to read aloud.

Welcome to the sexual health in recovery group. We are here to talk about sex and how our sexual lives affect recovery from drug and alcohol addiction. Some people in recovery risk a relapse because of their sexual behavior at the treatment center or away from the treatment program. This is a place to talk about sexual behavior and sexual health so we can be abstinent from drugs and alcohol. It is also a place to learn about sexual behavior and situations that put men and women in recovery at risk for not completing this treatment program.

Sexual health in recovery is a time to talk about human sexuality and sexual health in a respectful and informed manner. We encourage everyone to be as honest and open as you can be. You are not required to reveal anything about your current or past sexual behavior that would be uncomfortable to discuss. It is important to listen to each other. For some of us, our sexual behavior is the most serious risk to staying in recovery. For others, our sexual behavior gets us into dangerous situations that are triggers to use or drink. A few of us may have little concern about how our sexual behavior contributes to relapse. This group is an opportunity for everyone to learn about the important connection between recovery and sexual health.

LESSON INTRODUCTION

Ask another group member to volunteer to read aloud.

The purpose of today's sexual health in recovery group is to discuss motivations for sex and how our motivations for sex will increase or decrease our chances for staying sober. We will learn exciting new research on over 100 different motivations for sex. We will learn how men and women are similar and different in their motivations for sex. Sexual health in recovery believes that men and women in recovery need to take time for honest reflection about current motivations for sex. Today we will create several decks of cards to demonstrate the various motivations for sex. We will learn 50 sexual motivations commonly linked with drug/alcohol addiction. We will play a Family Feud game format using recent sex research surveys to talk about motivations for sex. The "I STILL Want to Have Sex in Recovery Worksheet" will be utilized as a relapse prevention skill to pause and reflect on motivations for sex in recovery.

LECTURE

Leader: What motivates humans to have sex? We are going to find out today that it may not be as simple a question as we assume. For some people the only motivation for sex is to reproduce. For others it may be for pleasure. Some may be motivated to have sex to express love or affection for someone. Other times it may be as practical, such as a relief from tension.

New sex research from the University of Texas has expanded our understanding of the reasons people have sex (Meston & Buss, 2007). The study found that the reasons people have sex are much more psychologically complex than just procreation, expression of love, and tension release. The exercises we are going to do today will increase our understanding of just how complex motivations for sex can be when addiction is combined with these motivations. We will focus on understanding the sexual motives that are typical among men and women with addictions. Sexual health in recovery includes understanding that humans have a very wide range of motivations for sex.

EXPERIENTIAL LEARNING

Leader: The University of Texas researchers found over 200 reasons why people have sex. They found that all of these reasons could be organized into four broad categories: our bodies, our emotions, our goals, and our insecurities. To learn about each of these four motivation categories, we are going to put together decks of index cards. We have four colors of index cards: green, red, purple, and white. We are going to make these colored index cards into sexual health decks that we will use to better understand women's and men's similar and different motivations for sex. First, let's divide into two working groups.

Divide the class evenly into two groups, A and B. The groups do not need to be divided by gender. (The exercise will work no matter what the configuration of the two groups, even if all clients are of the same gender.) Wait for the groups to form before giving further instructions.

Leader: Group A is going to help us learn about top 50 motivations for sexual intercourse among women. Group B is going to help us learn about the top 50 motivations for sexual intercourse among men.

Hand out a deck of colored cards, scissors, and tape to each group. Give Group A the list of 50 reasons women have sexual intercourse from "Why Humans Have Sex" (Meston & Buss, 2007) (Lesson 4 appendix, A). Give Group B the list of the 50 reasons men have sexual intercourse from the same research (Lesson 4 appendix, B) Have the lists in sealed envelopes to avoid distraction before beginning the exercise.

Leader: Group A has a list of the 50 motivations for why women have sexual intercourse. Group B has the list of the 50 motivations for why men have sexual intercourse from the same research.

Do not open the envelopes with the lists until directed. Remember the four broad categories of motivations for sex we just discussed? Who can remind the group of those four general categories?

Review the four categories of body, emotions, goals, and insecurities. Have a PowerPoint slide showing the four categories and their corresponding colors.

Leader: As you can see on the screen

■ Green is for the body-focused motivations for sex,
■ Red is for emotion-focused motivations for sex,
■ White is for goal-focused motivations for sex, and
■ Purple is for insecurity-focused motivations for sex.

Leader: On the screen is a sample of the list in your envelope. You will notice that the description of the reason is labeled with the corresponding general motivation category and the color.

A sample slide might appear like this:
    It just happened (BODY-GREEN)
    I want to increase the emotional bond by having sex (EMOTION-RED)

Leader: The task of each group is to take the lists you have in your envelopes and cut out each motivation, match it with the correct color card, and tape it to the appropriately colored card. There will be a few motivations that are duplicated because they are a combination of two categories; make two cards for these motivations and include the motivation in both colors of cards.

Group A will write "Women" on the front of every card. Group B will write "Men" on the front of every card.

While each group is completing the task, I encourage you to discuss among group members any thoughts or observations you are having about the list. This is not a time for personal disclosure of your sex life. It is a time to discuss what you think about the information. Are you surprised by what is on the list? Are you unsure what a particular motivation means? Ask your fellow group members what they think the motivation may mean. This is not a time to focus on what would be *your* top 50 motivations. There will be time later in the class when you will get a chance to focus on how this information relates to you. So keep your focus on the list and accomplishing your task. Have fun. We have about 10–15 minutes to complete this task. Any questions?

> *Direct groups to open their envelopes. Let each group figure out how to accomplish the task. This is part of the experience of finding a way to work together. Facilitate the exercise by supporting each group in task completion, answering questions, and keeping each group focused on the task. Give time cues so groups know how to pace their activity. At the end of the activity lead a brief discussion on what it was like for each group to complete this task. Have group A and B stay seated together for this discussion.*

Leader: You may be surprised to learn what the researchers learned. Twenty of the top 25 motivations for sexual intercourse were the same for men and for women. The order of importance was somewhat different between men and women, but 20 of the top 25 most frequent motivations for sexual intercourse were the same.

However, men's motivations were much more frequently reported to center on physical appearance and physical desire. This supports the idea that men tend to be sexually aroused by visual cues. Men also reported higher motivations for seeking sexual experiences and more frequent opportunities for sex. This would lead to the men's deck of motivations perhaps having more green cards.

Have a member of Group B count the number of green cards in their stack. Have a member of Group A count the green cards in their stack. See if their findings correspond with the research.

Leader: On the other hand, women reported a much higher frequency of emotional motivations for sex.

Have group members count the number of red cards in the Group A's deck compared to Group B's deck; see if their findings correspond with the research.

Leader: Men also were motivated to have sexual intercourse as a means of increasing their social status. This is a goal of sex that is more frequent among men than women. This would be white cards. Men will be motivated to accomplish the goal of increasing their status among their friends or social group.

Have groups A and group B remain seated together and move to the next exercise.

Leader: When it comes to the most common motivations for sexual intercourse, it turns out that men and women may have much more in common with each other than they have differences. What are some motivations for sex among addicts? What might their motivations for sex look like when they are beginning recovery? I have a deck of index cards similar to the two you just created in your groups. Each card lists one sex/drug-linked motivation for sex. These cards comprise 50 high-frequency motivations for sex that are more common during active addiction.

Take out the premade deck of Sexual Motivations in Addiction cards.

Leader: This is called sexual motivations in addiction. We are going to use this deck to see what playing with sexual motivations highly linked with addiction looks like. First, let's go back to the four broad motivation categories for sexual intercourse.

Return to the PowerPoint slide with the four categories and corresponding colors. Ask the group to think about which colors may be more frequent in the sexual health deck. To demonstrate this, have a volunteer come to the front of the room and organize the sexual motivations in addiction cards by color into four stacks. Have the volunteer hand the stack of white cards (goal-focused motivations) to group A. Hand purple cards (insecurity motivations) to Group B.

Ask members of Group A to read aloud the motivation statements on each of their cards. Have the group listen quietly. Then have the members of Group B do the same with their cards. What will be clearly obvious is that the sexual motivations in addiction cards are almost exclusively purple and white.

Compare the number of red and green cards in the sexual motivations in addiction deck to the 50 most common sexual motivations for men and for women decks. Then compare the number of white and purple cards in the sexual motivations in addiction deck to the other two decks. Have group discuss thoughts and reactions to this information.

When the discussion is complete, hand out the list of "50 Sex/Drug-Linked Motivations for Sexual Intercourse" (Lesson 4 appendix, C) to each group member.

Leader: This is a list of 50 sex/drug-linked motivations for sexual intercourse. All 50 of these items are not in either men's or women's top 50 motivations for having sexual intercourse. Many of these motivations may be more frequent among people who have become addicted to drugs or alcohol. A few of these motivations may *only* occur among people in recovery. These motivations are difficult to be honest about.

Almost every one of these motivations is reported in sex research that studies motivations for sex. Although these motivations are much less frequent, they carry much greater negative and harmful consequences, particularly for individuals who are addicted to drugs and alcohol. Just because they are less common motivations does not mean they are less important. The individuals who endure the harmful and hurtful consequences of these sexual motivations are also found in very high percentages among men and women in treatment. This is a very important reason why understanding sex/drug-linked sexuality is so important in improving treatment outcomes.

A sexual health in recovery goal is to honestly evaluate your motivations for sex and assess which of your motivations may be highly linked with using drugs and alcohol. This is why you should keep this list and use as much as you need for your recovery.

TOPIC SKILL PRACTICE

Leader: Now for some fun. Who remembers the game show Family Feud?

Have participants describe the television game show and how it works. Emphasize that people work in small family teams or groups to answer questions about survey results about certain human behaviors or opinions. The goal is to find the most frequently given answers by people filling out the survey.

Leader: Thanks for the explanation. We are going to play a brief version of this game using information from the surveys given to the men and women in the motivations for sex survey.

Have participants divide into groups of 3–5 teams, depending on the size of the class. Ideally each team will have 4–5 members. The task of each team is to answer survey questions when it is their turn. The questions and correct answers can be put into a PowerPoint presentation, which can be used for revealing each correct answer (see Lesson 4 appendix, D, for a list of questions and answers). Sounds may be used for identifying correct or incorrect answers if possible. This keeps spontaneity, humor, and fun in each survey response.

Leader: We're going to play the game like Family Feud. I'm going to ask a question, and each group has 3 minutes to come up with an answer they believe will be on the list of survey responses from the research on motivations for sex. Each team should appoint a spokesperson to give the answer for the team. Each team has time to debate and discuss the answer before the spokesperson gives the answer. If one team gives a wrong answer, I will move onto the next team.

While the game is being played, give feedback to the other teams who are thinking, sharing and discussing their answers. They need to be prepared to answer should the current team's guess be incorrect. This group process will prepare group members for the upcoming portion of the I STILL Want to Have Sex in Recovery Worksheet where they consider motivations for sex and discuss them with their support system. Play as many of the survey questions as time allows. (See Lesson 4 appendix, D, for questions and survey answers. Facilitators can go directly to the source material research to create additional survey questions. Time permitting, play at least two rounds of survey responses.)
Have participants return to their seats for the last section of the lesson. Hand out the I STILL Want to Have Sex in Recovery Worksheet.

Leader: This worksheet will focus on using our newfound information about why humans have sex. Notice the section where you consider your motivations for sex that may be sex/drug linked and those that may not be sex/drug linked. You can use the handouts on the top 50 motivations for men and for women to have sex as well as the sex/drug-linked motivations for sex to assist you in filling out this form. By making up the index card decks and playing the Family Feud game, you have all had some experience with talking to others in recovery about motivations for sex. Congratulations, you have all just completed some very important skill building for sexual health in recovery.

CLOSING

Leader: Let's take a moment to prepare for ending this sexual health in recovery session. Take a deep breath to quiet your mind, your heart, and your spirit. In this quiet place, remind yourself how valuable it is to take the time to be honest, vulnerable, and committed to sexual health in recovery. As you leave the group today, remind yourself that a satisfying sexual life is a vital and important part of recovery. The self-reflection and tools you learned today may become an important part of maintaining your recovery.

REFERENCES

Johnson, K. (1997). *Human sexual motivation.* Retrieved December 12, 2008, from http://www.csun.edu/~vcpsy00h/students/sexmotiv.htm

Meston, C., & Buss, D. (2007). Why humans have sex. *Archives of Sexual Behavior, 36,* 477–507.

Ott, M., Millstein, S., Ofner, S., & Halpern-Fisher, B. (2006). Greater expectations: Adolescents' positive motivations for sex. *Perspectives on Sexual and Reproductive Health, 38*(2), 84–89.

LESSON 4 APPENDIX

A. 50 Most Frequent Reasons Women Have Sexual Intercourse

Body: GREEN (stress reduction, pleasure, physical desirability, experience seeking)

Emotions: RED (love and commitment, expression of emotions)

Goals: WHITE (resources, revenge, status)

Insecurity: PURPLE (self-esteem boost, duty/pressure, mate guarding)

1. I am attracted to the person (BODY-GREEN)
2. I want to experience the physical pleasure (BODY-GREEN)
3. It feels good (BODY-GREEN)
4. I want to show my affection to the person (EMOTION-RED)
5. I want to express my love for the person (EMOTION-RED)
6. I am sexually aroused and want the release (BODY-GREEN)
7. I am horny (BODY-GREEN)
8. It's fun (BODY-GREEN)
9. I realized I am in love (EMOTION-RED)
10. The heat of the moment (BODY-GREEN)
11. I want to please my partner (BODY-GREEN and EMOTION-RED)
12. I desire emotional closeness and intimacy (EMOTION-RED)
13. I want the pure pleasure (BODY-GREEN)
14. I want to achieve an orgasm (BODY-GREEN)
15. It's exciting and adventurous (BODY-GREEN)
16. I want to feel connected to the person (EMOTION-RED)
17. The person's physical appearance turned me on (BODY-GREEN)
18. It is a romantic setting (BODY-GREEN and EMOTION-RED)
19. The person really desired me (BODY-GREEN and EMOTION-RED)
20. The person made me feel sexy (BODY-GREEN and EMOTION-RED)
21. The person caressed me (BODY-GREEN and EMOTION-RED)
22. It seemed like the natural next step in my relationship (EMOTION-RED)

23. I wanted to become one with another person (EMOTION-RED)
24. It just happened (BODY-GREEN)
25. I want to increase the emotional bond by having sex (EMOTION-RED)
26. I want the experience (BODY-GREEN)
27. I want the adventure/excitement (BODY-GREEN)
28. The person had an attractive face (BODY-GREEN)
29. The person was a good kisser (BODY-GREEN and EMOTION-RED)
30. I want to intensify my relationship (EMOTION-RED)
31. My hormones were out of control (none of the four)
32. I want to try out new sexual techniques or positions (BODY-GREEN)
33. I want to feel loved (EMOTION-RED and INSECURITY-PURPLE)
34. The person had a desirable body (BODY-GREEN)
35. I wanted to celebrate birthday, anniversary, special occasion (EMOTION-RED)
36. I want to communicate at a deeper level (EMOTION-RED)
37. I was curious about sex (BODY-GREEN)
38. It was a special occasion (BODY-GREEN and EMOTION-RED)
39. The person is intelligent (BODY-GREEN and EMOTION-RED)
40. I want to say "I miss you" (EMOTION-RED)
41. I want to keep my partner satisfied (EMOTION-RED))
42. I got carried away (BODY-GREEN and INSECURITY-PURPLE)
43. The opportunity presented itself (BODY-GREEN)
44. The person had a great sense of humor (BODY-GREEN and EMOTION-RED)
45. I want to improve my sexual skills (BODY-GREEN)
46. I was curious about my sexual abilities (BODY-GREEN)
47. The person seemed self-confident (BODY-GREEN AND EMOTION-RED)
48. I want to make up after a fight (none of the four)
49. I was drunk (BODY-GREEN)
50. I was turned on by the sexual conversation (BODY-GREEN)

Adapted from Meston and Buss (2007, pp. 481–482).

B. 50 Most Frequent Reasons Men Have Sexual Intercourse

Body: GREEN (stress reduction, pleasure, physical desirability, experience seeking)

Emotions: RED (love and commitment, expression of emotions)

Goals: WHITE (resources, revenge, status)

Insecurity: PURPLE (self-esteem boost, duty/pressure, mate guarding)

1. I am attracted to the person (BODY-GREEN)
2. It feels good (BODY-GREEN)
3. I want to experience the physical pleasure (BODY-GREEN)
4. It's fun (BODY-GREEN)
5. I want to show my affection to the person (EMOTION-RED)
6. I am sexually aroused and want the release (BODY-GREEN)
7. I am horny (BODY-GREEN)
8. I want to express my love for the person (EMOTION-RED)
9. I want to achieve an orgasm (BODY-GREEN)
10. I want to please my partner (BODY-GREEN and EMOTION-RED)
11. The person's physical appearance turned me on (BODY-GREEN)
12. I want the pure pleasure (BODY-GREEN)
13. The heat of the moment (BODY-GREEN)
14. I desire emotional closeness and intimacy (EMOTION-RED)
15. It's exciting and adventurous (BODY-GREEN)
16. The person had a desirable body (BODY-GREEN)
17. I realized I am in love (EMOTION-RED)
18. The person has an attractive face (BODY-GREEN)
19. The person really desired me (BODY-GREEN and EMOTION-RED)
20. I want the adventure/excitement (BODY-GREEN)
21. I want to feel connected to the person (EMOTION-RED)
22. I want the experience (BODY-GREEN)
23. It is a romantic setting (BODY-GREEN and EMOTION-RED)
24. The person caressed me (BODY-GREEN and EMOTION-RED)

25. The person made me feel sexy (BODY-GREEN and EMOTION-RED)
26. It seemed like the natural next step in my relationship (EMOTION-RED)
27. I want to increase the emotional bond by having sex (EMOTION-RED)
28. I want to keep my partner satisfied (EMOTION-RED)
29. The opportunity presented itself (BODY-GREEN)
30. It just happened (BODY-GREEN)
31. I want to intensify the relationship (EMOTION-RED)
32. I want to try out new sexual techniques or positions (BODY-GREEN)
33. My hormones were out of control (none of the four)
34. The person was too hot (sexy) to resist (BODY-GREEN)
35. I was curious about my sexual abilities (BODY-GREEN)
36. I want to improve my sexual skills (BODY-GREEN)
37. I wanted to become one with another person (EMOTION-RED)
38. I saw the person naked and could not resist (BODY-GREEN)
39. The person was a good kisser (BODY-GREEN and EMOTION-RED)
40. I want to feel loved (EMOTION-RED and INSECURITY-PURPLE)
41. I wanted to celebrate birthday, anniversary, special occasion (EMOTION-RED)
42. The person was too physically attractive to resist (BODY-GREEN)
43. It was a special occasion (BODY-GREEN and EMOTION-RED)
44. I hadn't had sex in a while (BODY-GREEN)
45. The person had beautiful eyes (BODY-GREEN)
46. I want to communicate at a deeper level (EMOTION-RED)
47. I want to experiment with a new experience (BODY-GREEN)
48. The person is intelligent (BODY-GREEN and EMOTION-RED)
49. I want to keep my partner happy (INSECURITY-PURPLE and EMOTION-RED)
50. I was curious what the person was like in bed (BODY-GREEN)

Adapted from Meston and Buss (2007, pp. 481–482).

C. 50 Sex/Drug-Linked Motivations for Sexual Intercourse

All 50 of these motivations for sexual intercourse are not in either men or women's top 50 motivations for having sexual intercourse. Many of these motivations may be more frequent among people who have become addicted to drugs or alcohol. A few of these motivations may only occur among people in recovery. These motivations are difficult to be honest about. Almost every one of these motivations is reported in sex research that studies motivations for sex. The goal for sexual health in recovery is to honestly evaluate your motivations for sex and assess what motivations for sex are low and which motivations are too often linked with drugs and alcohol.

Body: GREEN (stress Reduction, pleasure, physical desirability, experience seeking)

Emotions: RED (love and commitment, expression of emotions)

Goals: WHITE (resources, revenge, status)

Insecurity: PURPLE (self-esteem boost, duty/pressure, mate guarding)

1. I want to give someone a sexually transmitted disease (e.g., herpes, HIV) (GOALS-WHITE)
2. The person offered to give me drugs for doing it (GOALS-WHITE)
3. Someone offered me money to do it (GOALS-WHITE)
4. I want to break up my relationship (GOALS-WHITE)
5. It was an initiation rite to a club or gang (GOALS-WHITE)
6. I want to punish myself (GOALS-WHITE)
7. I was afraid to say "no" because of the possibility of physical harm (GOALS-WHITE)
8. I want to hurt/humiliate the person (GOALS-WHITE)
9. I want to make money (GOALS-WHITE)
10. I want to break up another person's relationship (GOALS-WHITE)
11. I want to get a favor from someone (GOALS-WHITE)
12. I want to be used or degraded (GOALS-WHITE)
13. I want to hurt an enemy (GOALS-WHITE)

14. I want to get back at my partner for having cheated on me (GOALS-WHITE)
15. I was physically forced to (INSECURITY-PURPLE)
16. It was a favor to someone (GOALS-WHITE)
17. The person had too much to drink and I was able to take advantage of them (GOALS-WHITE)
18. I want to get even with someone (GOALS-WHITE)
19. I want to make someone jealous (GOALS-WHITE)
20. I want to manipulate him/her into doing something for me (INSECURITY-PURPLE)
21. My partner kept on insisting (INSECURITY-PURPLE)
22. I was competing with someone to get the person (GOALS-WHITE)
23. I am addicted to sex (BODY-GREEN)
24. I want to have sex while stoned or high (BODY-GREEN)
25. I was drunk (BODY-GREEN)
26. I am a sex addict (BODY-GREEN)
27. I wanted to satisfy a compulsion (BODY-GREEN)
28. The person wore revealing clothes (BODY-GREEN)
29. I was concerned about getting turned on (BODY-GREEN)
30. I want to lose my inhibitions (BODY-GREEN)
31. I want to have more sex than friends or other couples do (GOALS-WHITE)
32. The person is famous and I want to be able to say I had sex with him/her (GOALS-WHITE)
33. I want to relapse and have a good excuse (INSECURITY-PURPLE)
34. I want to impress my friends (GOALS-WHITE)
35. I am on the rebound from another relationship (GOALS-WHITE)
36. I want to keep my partner satisfied (EMOTIONS-RED and INSECURITY-PURPLE)
37. It is taboo and forbidden in the recovery community (INSECURITY-PURPLE)
38. I am afraid to have sex sober (INSECURITY-PURPLE)
39. I want to put passion back in my relationship (EMOTIONS-RED)
40. I want to put passion back in my relationship (INSECURITY-PURPLE)
41. I want to boost my self-esteem (INSECURITY-PURPLE)

42. I feel rebellious (INSECURITY-PURPLE)
43. I want to feel closer to God (GOALS-WHITE)
44. I want to possess the person (GOALS-WHITE))
45. I don't know how to say "no" (INSECURITY-PURPLE)
46. My partner kept insisting (INSECURITY-PURPLE)
47. I physically forced my partner without consent (INSECURITY-PURPLE)
48. I was physically forced to without my consent (INSECURITY-PURPLE)
49. I want to keep my partner from leaving me (INSECURITY-PURPLE)
50. I want the person to love me (INSECURITY-PURPLE)

Adapted from Meston and Buss (2007, pp. 493–495).

D. Family Feud Game Survey Questions

Have a PowerPoint slide with each question displayed on the screen. Have slides indicating whether an answer is "Correct" or "Incorrect" (with appropriate audio, if possible). The top 10 correct answers, as well as 5 incorrect answers, are listed below.

Survey Question 1: What are the 10 *least* frequent motivations for sex reported by both men and women?

Correct Answers
1. I wanted to give someone else a sexually transmitted disease (e.g., herpes, AIDS).
2. The person offered to give me drugs for doing it.
3. Someone offered me money to do it.
4. I wanted to get a raise.
5. I wanted to punish myself.
6. I wanted to break up my relationship.
7. I wanted to get a job.
8. I was afraid to say "no" because of the possibility of physical harm.
9. I wanted to hurt/humiliate the person.
10. I wanted to feel closer to God.

Incorrect Answers
1. I wanted to see what it would be like to have sex while stoned (e.g., on marijuana or some other drug).
2. I wanted to get back at my partner for having cheated on me.
3. I wanted to avoid hurting someone's feelings.
4. The person had too much to drink and I was able to take advantage of them.
5. I was under the influence of drugs.

Survey Question 2: What are the top 10 motivations reported by men for having sex?

Correct Answers
1. I was attracted to the person.
2. It feels good.
3. I wanted to experience the physical pleasure.
4. It's fun.

5. I wanted to show my affection for the person.
6. I was sexually aroused and wanted the release.
7. I was horny.
8. I wanted to express my love for the person.
9. I wanted to achieve an orgasm.
10. I wanted to please my partner.

Incorrect Answers
1. I was in the heat of the moment.
2. The person had too much to drink and I was able to take advantage of them.
3. The person demanded that I have sex with him/her.
4. I saw the person naked and could not resist.
5. I hadn't had sex in a while.

Survey Question 3: What are the top 10 motivations reported by women for having sex?

Correct Answers
1. I was attracted to the person.
2. I wanted to experience the physical pleasure.
3. It feels good.
4. I wanted to show my affection for the person.
5. I wanted to express my love for the person.
6. I was sexually aroused and wanted the release.
7. I was horny.
8. It's fun.
9. I realized I was in love.
10. I was in the heat of the moment.

Incorrect Answers
1. It just happened.
2. I wanted to feel loved.
3. I was drunk.
4. My hormones were out of control.
5. The person was a good kisser.

Survey Question 4: According to a recent survey, what are the five most frequent motivations for insecure men and women to have sex?

Correct Answers

1. I felt insecure.
2. I felt like it was my duty.
3. I felt obligated to.
4. I didn't know how to say no.
5. I didn't want to disappoint the person.

Incorrect Answers

1. I wanted the person to love me.
2. I wanted to feel loved.
3. I wanted to feel powerful.
4. I wanted to raise my self-esteem.
5. I was physically forced to.

E. I STILL Want to Have Sex in Recovery Worksheet

There are five steps in STILL
  1. Stop
  2. Think
  3. Inform
  4. Listen
  5. Listen

This worksheet is a guide for what to do after you stop an impulse or urge before taking action. If you are reading this worksheet instead of acting impulsively, congratulations, you chose to stop and think.

> Think: The thinking step involves identifying sex/drug-linked motivations for sex and non-sex/drug-linked motivations for sex by rating their risk for relapse.

Take out the list of the top 50 motivations for sex for either men or women. Take out the list of the top 50 sex/drug-linked motivations for sex.

> Write down up to five sex/drug-linked motivations for this current potential sexual situation. Items can be from the lists or your own thoughts.
>
>   1. _____
>
>   2. _____
>
>   3. _____
>
>   4. _____
>
>   5. _____

Write down up to five non-sex/drug-linked motivations. Items can be from the lists or your own thoughts.

  1. _____

  2. _____

  3. _____

4. _____

5. _____

Stop and think for a moment and then rate which motivation is the highest risk for relapse. Write it here. _____

Stop and think for a moment and then rate which motivation is the most consistent with recovery and sobriety. Write it here.

_____

When you have completed this section go to the next step: Inform.

Inform: Take your answers and inform a key trusted member of your support system. Do not talk with the person with whom you are having the sexual feelings or interest to complete this step. Inform your key support person of your sexual situation and motivations.

Listen: Have him/her listen to your written responses that you filled out about motivations for sex. The job of your support person is to first listen to your responses. He or she should listen without interruption and concentrate on hearing your thoughts and assessment of the situation. This is the part where you are listened to.

Listen: The last step is to listen to what your key support person says after listening to you. This is your time to listen without interruption. The key to this skill is to listen. Listening does not mean agreement. Listening does not mean complying. Listening is a form of concentration with the focus on paying attention to what another person is saying. Listening is an effort to hear and take into account what your key support person is saying.

The ability to stop, think, inform, and listen will be a significant skill in improving sexual health in recovery.

5 Talking about Sexual Health

CORE CONCEPT

Drug and alcohol dependent clients all too often withhold discussing their sexual health worries and problems because they fear their own judgment as well as judgmental responses from professional helpers, sponsors, or fellow clients. Sexual health in recovery is the ability to suspend judgmental thoughts and reactions to enable a more honest and open discussion about sexuality. Participants will learn self-observation skills to hear their own disapproving thoughts that interfere with honest self-disclosure. Being able to identify and temporarily turn down negative thoughts is a vital sexual health skill. We will practice setting aside—suspending—critical or rigid judgments to discuss highly emotionally charged sexual situations, behaviors, and thoughts related to recovery. We will learn how to use the "Suspending My Judgmental Thoughts and Behavior Worksheet" recovery tool (Lesson 5 appendix). Participants will practice suspending judgmental thoughts by hanging them on a clothesline. We will use role-play situations to practice talking about sex and suspending judgment of self and others.

BELIEF STATEMENT

Sexual health in recovery is the ability to suspend judgmental thoughts and reactions to enable a more honest and open discussion about sexuality.

OBJECTIVES

Participants will
- Explore how judgmental thoughts and statements interfere with sexual health discussions in recovery.
- Utilize experiential exercises to practice setting aside critical or rigid judgments to discuss highly emotionally charged sexual situations, behaviors, and thoughts related to recovery.
- Learn how to use the "Suspending My Judgmental Thoughts and Behavior Worksheet" sexual health in recovery tool.

CHANGE GOALS

- Increase knowledge of useful attitudes for exploring sexuality in recovery.
- Increase thinking and behavior patterns that support self-exploration of sexuality.
- Use the "Suspending My Judgmental Thoughts and Behavior Worksheet" recovery tool for exploring sexuality.

REQUIRED READING FOR GROUP LEADER

The key skill for the group leader and participants is to suspend judgmental thinking and behavior. What does a conversation where judgmental thoughts and behaviors are suspended look like? To answer this question, facilitators need to read a detailed deconstruction of suspension of judgmental thoughts and behavior.

Facilitators should begin with *Dialogue* by James C. Clawson (2008) from the University of Virginia–Darden Graduate School of Business Administration. This is an online case and teaching paper series located on the Internet at the award-winning Social Science Research

Network. On page 6, Clawson delineates judging from suspension in clear and precise terms. Page 9 reviews a range of dialogue techniques, some of which are practiced in this lesson. Although Clawson's material was written for a business setting, the content about suspending judgment is essential knowledge for leaders to facilitate this lesson.

RECOMMENDED MATERIALS FOR GROUP LEADER

Dialectical behavioral therapy (DBT) is a cognitive-behavioral psychotherapy for men and women with substantial and inflexible personality patterns that lead to a wide range of emotional, relational, and behavioral problems. Men and women with these rigid personality patterns pose significant treatment challenges. Core mindfulness skills are one of four key learned DBT skills used to decrease destructive personality behaviors. There are similarities between suspending judgment and mindfulness. Facilitators of this lesson will profit from expanding their repertoire of suspending judgmental responses and modeling this behavior for group members. The following DBT resources are recommended:

- www.DBTSelfHelp.com (Dietz, 2003) is a Web site for people seeking information about DBT. See, in particular, the lesson on *Nonjudgmental Stance*. The "Suspending My Judgmental Thoughts and Behavior Worksheet" is based on the same sequence of nonjudgmental steps presented there. Clients may want to explore www.DBTselfhelp.com. The site is very user friendly and written for the general public. It is not a drug and alcohol treatment site. This may normalize many thinking patterns (so-called stinking thinking) that addicts may assume are unique or specific to recovery.
- Tara Guest Arnold (2008), PhD, LCSW, wrote *Dialectical Behavior Therapy (DBT): Core Mindfulness* to summarize the technical skills for improving nonjudgmental mindfulness.
- In Marsha Linehan's groundbreaking 1993 text, *Cognitive-Behavioral Treatment of Borderline Personality Disorder*, core mindfulness psychological and behavioral skills are well defined and described on pages 144–147 (Linehan, 1993).

REQUIRED MATERIALS FOR THE LESSON

- An mp3 player and music selection
- Blackboard, white board, or flip chart
- Clothesline (hang clothesline from one side of room to the other at shoulder height before class begins)
- Clothes pins for each participant
- Blank 3 × 5 index cards
- Copies of "Suspending My Judgmental Thoughts and Behavior Worksheet" (one copy for each participant) (Lesson 5 appendix)

OPENING

Opening Music: *Have quiet music playing as participants enter the room and ready themselves (optional).*

Leader: As we sit quietly and focus on being here, let us clear our minds of where we have been and focus on being in this moment.

Opening Poem/Reading:

But how do we navigate the mysteries of sex?
We say we are swept away possessed and overtaken—
All of which acknowledge the force of desire but never its logic.
Is it possible to develop a kind of sexual intelligence,
one that can deepen our pleasure
and give us a greater awareness of ourselves?

—Kim Cattrall, *Sexual Intelligence* (2005)

GROUP INTRODUCTION

Have a group member volunteer to read aloud.

Welcome to the sexual health in recovery group. We are here to talk about sex and how our sexual lives affect recovery from drug and alcohol addiction. Some people in recovery risk a relapse because of their sexual behavior at the treatment center or away from the treatment program. This is a place to talk about sexual behavior and sexual health so we can be abstinent from drugs and alcohol. It is also a place to learn about sexual behavior and situations that put men and women in recovery at risk for not completing this treatment program.

Sexual health in recovery is a time to talk about human sexuality and sexual health in a respectful and informed manner. We encourage everyone to be as honest and open as you can be. You are not required to reveal anything about your current or past sexual behavior that would be uncomfortable to discuss. It is important to listen to each other. For some of us, our sexual behavior is the most serious risk to staying in recovery. For others, our sexual behavior gets us into dangerous situations that are triggers to use or drink. A few of us may have little concern about how our sexual behavior contributes to relapse. This group is an opportunity for everyone to learn about the important connection between recovery and sexual health.

LESSON INTRODUCTION

Ask another group member to volunteer to read aloud.

The purpose of today's sexual health in recovery group is to learn some basic skills for talking about our sexual lives to increase our chances to stay sober and in recovery. Recovering women and men will increase their likelihood of staying sober when they learn how to suspend judgmental sexual attitudes and behavior. Having sex-positive language and a nonjudgmental space for exploring sexual attitudes and values is an important sexual health skill for recovery.

We will identify attitudes that reduce feeling afraid and anxious about exploring sexuality in recovery. We will learn how to suspend some of our critical or rigid judgments in order to think or talk about our sexual desires and values. We will identify common thoughts and behaviors that create emotionally charged judgments about sex. We will practice a few tools to improve our skills in discussing sexuality. You will learn behaviors to improve your effectiveness in discussing sexuality in recovery.

LECTURE

Leader: Talking about sexuality, whether our own or that of others, can be filled with emotions. Sometimes discussing the topic of sexuality can make us feel full of curiosity, fascination, and even pleasurable excitement. Other times we may feel anxious, worried, embarrassed, and ashamed. Sexuality is so complex and full of self-meaning that it can feel overwhelming to even approach the subject. What is very common for almost all adults is that talking about our sexuality in a respectful and informed manner is pretty rare. It may be even less common for men and women in early recovery to have accurate, informed, and relevant information about sexuality and sobriety. Today we will focus on talking about our sexual behavior, attitudes, and values and learn a skill to increase our open-mindedness about addressing sexuality.

Leader: One definition of *suspend* is: "To stop something or make something ineffective, usually for a short time." Another is: "To delay or defer an action on a decision or a judgment until more of the facts are known" (Encarta Encyclopedia, 2009a).

Judgment can be defined as "an opinion formed or decision reached in the case of a disputed, controversial, or doubtful manner" or as "The ability to form sound opinions and make sensible decisions or reliable guesses" (Encarta Encyclopedia, 2009b).

Does suspending judgment about sexuality mean abandoning all morals and rejecting your personal values? This is a very common mistaken idea, that if we suspend our judgments we must eliminate our values. The key here is to *suspend* our judgments. Take a break from our rigid beliefs. We are simply setting them aside just for the moment—not forgetting them, disowning them, or repudiating them. In this time-out space from judgments, we can see things we usually cannot see. This is the value of setting aside judgments to explore our sexual selves.

Gesture to clothesline, which should already be hung from one side of room to the other at shoulder height.

Leader: This clothesline represents this time-out space. We will hang our judgments on this line and then practice a few recovery-related discussions attempting to leave the judgments aside and focus on three skills. These three skills are:

1. Observe by listening without comment or interruption until the person is done saying what he or she needs to say.
2. Describe what you observed while listening. Let the person know you listened by describing only what you observed either in yourself or the other person. You will not say what you thought, your opinion, your advice, or your judgment.

3. Be present by staying in the moment, participating in the moment, and staying in the here and now by noticing what is happening. Ask yourself: How is what is happening right now a fact or situation that is related to sexual health in recovery and avoiding increased risk for sex/drug-linked relapse?

EXPERIENTIAL LEARNING

Leader: Now, we are going to discuss sexual topics that may lead to judgments.

On the board, write a list of sexual topics that adults in recovery may have on their mind. Such topics might include:

- *Attractions at AA/NA meetings*
- *Body image*
- *Having sober sex*
- *Masturbation*
- *Visualizing past drug use with former partners for fantasy during masturbation or sex*
- *Dealing with jealousy*
- *Secretive online sexual behavior*
- *Is chatting online with someone in a sex chat room having an affair?*
- *Pain during intercourse*
- *Disclosing a sexually transmitted infection*
- *Not feeling very sexual*
- *Is it possible to share too much information about sex?*
- *Sex is the only thing that makes me feel good*
- *Not wanting to have sex with a partner when he/she drinks*
- *Being in love with an ex-partner who is an addict*
- *How do I say what I want sexually with my partner when I am sober?*

Leader: Can you think of any other topics to add?

Have the group brainstorm a list of other sexual topics most likely to result in high emotions and strong judgments. This list can come from the list you wrote, as well as other topics from group members.

Hand out index cards. Have each group member write down a personal list of his or her top five high-emotion, high-judgment sex in recovery topics. (This list will be kept private and not shared with the group.)

Leader: Now, let's make a list of sexual behaviors or thoughts that are most likely to be a risk for relapse if not talked about openly and honestly.

Ask the group for their suggestions and write them on the board. The list may include:

- *Fantasizing about getting high and having sex while masturbating*
- *Inability to have sexual arousal sober*
- *Thinking you are turned on by the wrong things*
- *Feeling ashamed about what sexually arouses you*
- *History of nonconsensual sex when high (rape, forced sex with spouse, sexual contact with a child or teenager, exhibitionism, voyeurism, touching people without their permission)*
- *Having attractions or sexual feelings for someone of the same sex*
- *Meeting up with people online who are high or drunk*
- *Continuing to have a secret affair while married*
- *Downloading images of children or teenagers*
- *Self-induced vomiting to stay thin*
- *Planning to get high and have sex over the weekend*
- *Not being able to refuse someone who wants to have sex*
- *Having flashbacks of past sexual abuse*
- *Feeling shame about being with a violent or abusive partner*
- *Not knowing HIV status*
- *Being HIV positive and not telling anyone*
- *Taking money for sex*

Have each participant make a private list of his or her top five sexual topics that are most closely linked with using or relapse. They will not share this list with the group.

Leader: I want each of you to observe yourself while you are writing your list. Does your heart rate, breathing, or body temperature change? Are any memories coming to mind? What thoughts are on your mind? The key is to observe these events, not judge them as right or wrong or good or bad. The key task here is to notice without judgment.

Leader: The second part of suspending judgment is to describe what you observed.

Discuss the difference between a nonjudgmental and judgmental voice tone. You may wish to model the same sentence, said judgmentally and nonjudgmentally. Have several members of the group say a sentence both with nonjudgmental and judgmental tone. Have the group discuss what makes the difference between the two. Encourage the group to observe very small details in tone, body language, eye movement, and posture.

Leader: On your note cards, I want each of you to write your single most important sex/drug-linked relapse risk thought or behavior. It can be from the private list you wrote earlier, or a new one. Imagine you told your most trusted family member, friend, sponsor, counselor, or other professional helper what your wrote. Imagine the judgmental thought or behavior that you fear he or she would have. Write the judgment down on the card. Keep this to yourself. This is the skill of observing your judgments without reacting to them. You are just noticing the judgment as if you are watching a scene in a movie.

Use this experiential exercise as springboard for discussion about the necessity to know how to suspend judgments.

Leader: Now, we will do the clothesline exercise to practice the recovery tool of suspending judgment. When you are finished writing your judgment on the card, quietly walk up to the clothesline, fold your card in half with the writing on the inside, and use a clothespin to suspend the judgment.

Allow group members time to complete this exercise.

Leader: Now, let's make a list of common sex/drug relapse judgments men and women in recovery may say with their body language, speech, or thinking. What are some things people may say or do to indicate judgment?

Encourage the class to come up with examples of judgmental behaviors. Examples may be:

- *Interrupt to give an opinion*
- *Interrupt to give advice*
- *Make disgusted sounds or make disgusted facial expressions*
- *Laugh*
- *Snicker*
- *Express shock*
- *Make titillating or flirtatious comments*
- *Point out what is healthy or unhealthy*

- *Point out what is acceptable or unacceptable*
- *Assume the person may have a sexual addiction*
- *Immediately warn the person about the dangers of what he or she is doing*
- *Turn the focus on to yourself and share about your own sexual concerns*
- *Talk about what your religion, religious text, minister, church, or God thinks about the sexual behavior*

TOPIC SKILL PRACTICE

Leader: Let's review the three steps for nonjudgmental behavior: observe, describe, and be present.

Lead a discussion to review these three topics. Emphasize the following key concepts:

- *To observe is to notice without evaluation.*
- *Describe with facts of what is observed, not imagined or assumed.*
- *To be present is to focus on the moment, the feelings, the sensations, the experience of describing what is observed without commenting on the content of what was said. Being present also means to be aware of the sex/drug-linked relapse risk consequences of what was discussed, notice this, and then let it go.*

Leader: Now, we are going to role-play a discussion using one of the high risk for relapse sexual situations that would likely create a strong emotional reaction in both the listener and the speaker.

Ask two volunteers to role-play a 2–3 minute discussion using one of the high risk for relapse sexual situations that were discussed earlier and listed on the board. Ask one volunteer to be the speaker and one to be the listener. Have the speaker choose one of the sexual situations on the board and begin to speak about it. Coach the listener to pay attention and use the three-step approach to listening without judgment.

Before the role-play, hand out more blank cards to the rest of the group. Direct group members to notice their judgmental thoughts or behaviors while watching the role-play and write them down on the cards.

Sample role-play: Speaker discusses how she thinks of herself as a slut and can't forgive herself for all the sex she had when she was using. Listener notices what he/she is feeling, thinking, and observing about the speaker during the story. After a few minutes, the listener tells the speaker what he/she observed while listening. Then both participants share a few thoughts and feelings about what it is like to be present in this moment doing the role-play. Group members take their written judgments and suspend them on the clothesline after the role-play. Repeat as time permits.

Briefly process each role-play with a focus on what each person did well. You may praise the listener for his or her voice tone, facial expressions, and body language. You may praise the speaker for his or her use of clear factual words, avoidance of vague language, specificity, and use of clear details.

Ask observers to discuss alternative responses they thought of while watching the role-play.

Leader: Now I am going to hand out the "Suspending My Judgmental Thoughts and Behavior Worksheet" as a recovery tool. As we've done in class, this worksheet asks you to analyze a sexual behavior, thought, or action without judgment.

Hand out the "Suspending My Judgmental Thoughts and Behavior Worksheet" (Lesson 5 appendix) and explain it to the group.

CLOSING

Leader: Let's take a moment to prepare for ending this sexual health in recovery session. Take a deep breath to quiet your mind, your heart, and your spirit. In this quiet place, remind yourself how valuable it is to take the time to be honest, vulnerable, and committed to sexual health in recovery. As you leave the group today, remind yourself that sexual health in recovery includes knowing how to suspend your own judgments about sex and sexuality. Know also that the better you become at suspending judgment, the more open, honest, and proactive you can be about maintaining your recovery and preventing risk of relapse.

REFERENCES

Arnold T. G. (2008). *Dialectical behavior therapy (DBT): Core mindfulness.* Retrieved February 28, 2009, from http://www.goodtherapy.org/custom/blog/2008/01/23/dialectical-behavior-therapy-dbt-core-mindfulness/

Cattrall, K. (2005). *Sexual intelligence.* New York: Bullfinch Press.

Clawson, J. G. (2008). *Dialogue, 1,* pp. 1–16. Social Science Research Network. Retrieved May 24, 2009, from http://paper.ssrn.com/sol3/papers.cfm?abstract_id=910737

Dietz, L. (2003). *NonJudgemental stance.* DBT SelfHelp.org. Retrieved February 28, 2009, from http://www.dbtselfhelp.com/html/non-judgmental_stance.html

Encarta Encyclopedia. (2009a). Retrieved May 24, 2009, from http://encarta.msn.com/encnet/refpages/search.aspx?q=suspendAnother

Encarta Encyclopedia. (2009b). Retrieved May 24, 2009, from http://encarta.msn.com/encnet/refpages/search.aspx?q=Judgment

Linehan, M. (1993). *Cognitive-behavioral treatment of borderline personality disorder.* New York: The Guilford Press.

LESSON 5 APPENDIX

Suspending My Judgmental Thoughts and Behavior Worksheet

Suspending judgment is a vital skill for sexual health in recovery. It means learning to delay forming an opinion or judgment about a controversial sexual behavior, attitude, or thought.

Skills

- Observe the sex/drug-linked relapse risk that is on your mind.
- Describe what you notice about your thoughts and feelings when you think about this sex/drug-linked relapse risk. Notice the judgmental thoughts or reactions you have to this sex/drug-linked relapse risk.
- Suspend the judgment and notice how you feel and think when this judgment is suspended.
- Be present by staying in the moment, participating in the moment, and noticing what is happening. How is what is happening right now a fact or situation that is related to sexual health in recovery and avoiding increased risk for sex/drug-linked relapse?
- Take your judgment back when you are done suspending it.

Instructions: Write the sex/drug-linked relapse risk behavior, attitude, or thought that you are preparing to discuss.

_____

_____

_____

Make a check mark next to any of the judgmental behaviors you anticipate you may have about this sexual concern.

_____ Interrupt to give opinion or advice.

_____ Disgusted sounds or disgusted look on my face because I think it is immoral.

_____ Make confrontational, aggressive, and harsh comments.

_____ Look for evidence of delusions, impaired judgment, or denial and try to catch self-deception.

_____ Feel that I cannot be trustworthy or responsible in my sexual behavior.

_____ Laugh, snicker, or express shock.

_____ Say sexually titillating or flirtatious comments.

_____ Point out what is healthy and what is unhealthy sex.

_____ Expect everyone to agree with me about what is healthy or unhealthy sex.

_____ Assume I am a sex addict in denial.

_____ (Write a thought or belief not written here.)

_____

_____

_____

_____

Pick the judgment you are most concerned about experiencing with yourself or from others.

Write this judgment on a card or piece of paper.

Place this judgment in a suspended place (in a book, on a hanger in your closet, on the dashboard of your car, in your medicine cabinet, etc.).

Go about your day noticing when you think about this judgment. Remind yourself you have suspended this judgment for the day. Just be present with yourself and notice what it is like to remind yourself that you have suspended this judgment for today.

When you wake up the next day, take your suspended judgment back. Remember this is a skill about suspending judgment, not discarding or changing your judgment.

6

Spirituality and Sexuality in Recovery

CORE CONCEPT

In the course of their addiction, many women and men engage in a variety of sexual behaviors and situations that conflict with their individual spiritual and ethical values. Spiritual sexual health in recovery is not about religion and sex. Nor is it about exploring what your religion, faith, or sacred text says about sexuality. Spiritual sexual health in recovery encompasses the entire range of men and women's beliefs in God, from devout to nonbeliever. Spiritual sexual health combines ethical behavior with internationally respected global agreements of healthy sexual behavior.

Six fundamental principles of sexual health for all sexually active people form the foundation for women and men in recovery to understand their personal relapse risk consequences of sexual behavior that conflict with their ethics and values. The six principles are adapted from the World Health Organization (WHO) working definition of sexual health (WHO, 2006, p. 5) and *A Time to Speak: Faith Communities and Sexuality Education* list of "Healthy Sexual Relationships" (Haffner & Ott, 2005, p. 26). Theses principles provide an alternative to fearing sexuality as a relapse risk. Women and men in recovery increase their likelihood of staying sober when they connect universal principles of sexual health with their personal spiritual and ethical values.

Sexual health in recovery believes sexual behavior that is not grounded in universal principles of sexual health is a central risk for drinking or using. Using a deck of sex/drug-linked situation playing cards, participants will learn each principle and practice applying them in a variety of sexual situations. Participants will practice completing "The Sexuality and Spirituality in Recovery Inventory."

BELIEF STATEMENT

Sexual health in recovery is the ability to connect universal principles of sexual health with personal spiritual and ethical values.

OBJECTIVES

Participants will
- Learn about the tendency of men and women who have a significant pattern of devaluing or discounting the future to develop addictions.
- Learn six fundamentals of sexual health.
- Connect six fundamentals with building spirituality, ethics, and sexual health in recovery.
- Practice using the six principles of sexual health in a noncompetitive learning card game to challenge patterns of devaluing and discounting future concerns.
- Complete "The Sexuality and Spirituality in Recovery Inventory" (Lesson 6 appendix, B).

CHANGE GOALS

- Normalize high frequency of future devaluing defenses and perceptions among addicts and alcoholics.
- Understand the role of universal foundational principles of sexual health in developing ethical and spiritual sexuality in recovery.
- Utilize "The Sexuality and Spirituality in Recovery Inventory" (Lesson 6 appendix, B) to reinforce fundamentals of sexual health

in recovery and develop spirituality and ethical behavior within sexual activity.

REQUIRED READING FOR GROUP LEADER

Coleman, E. (2007). Sexual health and public policy: An introduction. *International Journal of Sexual Health, 19*(3), 1–24.

World Health Organization. (2006). *Defining sexual health: Report of a technical consultation on sexual health, 28–31 January 2002, Geneva.* Geneva, Switzerland: WHO Press.

Group leaders will develop an excellent overview of the history and development of current definitions of sexual health from these sources. This lesson is an integration of sexual health with spiritual principles. It will be the sexual health material in this lesson that may be new learning for most group leaders. It is vital for facilitators to have basic language, concepts, and definitions of sexual health to lead the discussions in this lesson.

RECOMMENDED MATERIALS FOR GROUP LEADER

Haffner, D., & Ott, K. (2005). *A time to speak: Faith communities and sexuality education programs, second edition* (online at www.religiousinstitute.org). This monograph advocates for "open and honest discourse about sexuality issues in faith communities" (p. 5) and the integration of sexual health education within faith communities throughout the lifespan. Consensual, non-exploitive, and mutually pleasurable components of healthy sexual relationships are listed on page 26. Group leaders will benefit from reading the "Denomination Statements About Sexuality Education" on pages 15–24. The authors list over a dozen different religious denominational resolutions that guide the sexuality education within each faith community.

Moore, T. (1998). *The soul of sex.* New York: HarperCollins. In chapter 8 (pp. 159–177) philosopher, writer, theologian, and former monk Thomas Moore explores the uncomfortable tension between moral principles and sexual desires. "In the midst of this moral anxiety and confusion, it is difficult to find sexual joy" (p. 160). Moore brings the language of sexual health within his discussion of basic sexual boundaries of conscience and erotic morality. "If we are feeling moralistic about some aspect of sex, sensing the need to limit sex in some way, the solution is not to overcome the inhibition but to take the lead of our feeling. We may find positive ways to diminish the importance of sex in relation to the rest of life. Demonizing what we need to limit only makes the complex more demanding and more negative" (p. 168).

REQUIRED MATERIALS FOR THE LESSON

- An mp3 player and music selection
- Blackboard, white board, or flip chart
- Deck of sex/drug-linked situation playing cards (see Lesson 6 appendix, A, for the terms on each playing card)
- Drawing of a compass with six directional points (directions will be filled in during the lesson)
- "The Sexuality and Spirituality in Recovery Inventory" (one copy for each participant) (Lesson 6 appendix, B)
- "List of Life Behaviors of a Sexually Healthy Adult" (Lesson 6 appendix, C)

OPENING

Opening Music: *Have quiet music playing as participants enter the room and ready themselves (optional).*

Leader: As we sit quietly and focus on being here, let us clear our minds of where we have been and focus on being in this moment.

Opening Poem/Reading:

We are not human beings having a spiritual experience. We are spiritual beings having a human experience.

—Pierre Teilhard de Chardin

GROUP INTRODUCTION

Have a group member volunteer to read aloud.

Welcome to the sexual health in recovery group. We are here to talk about sex and how our sexual lives affect recovery from drug and alcohol addiction. Some people in recovery risk a relapse because of their sexual behavior at the treatment center or away from the treatment program. This is a place to talk about sexual behavior and sexual health so we can be abstinent from drugs and alcohol. It is also a place to learn about sexual behavior and situations that put men and women in recovery at risk for not completing this treatment program.

Sexual health in recovery is a time to talk about human sexuality and sexual health in a respectful and informed manner. We encourage everyone to be as honest and open as you can be. You are not required to reveal anything about your current or past sexual behavior that would be uncomfortable to discuss. It is important to listen to each other. For some of us, our sexual behavior is the most serious risk to staying in recovery. For others, our sexual behavior gets us into dangerous situations that are triggers to use or drink. A few of us may have little concern about how our sexual behavior contributes to relapse. This group is an opportunity for everyone to learn about the important connection between recovery and sexual health.

LESSON INTRODUCTION

Ask another group member to volunteer to read aloud.

The purpose of today's sexual health in recovery group is to consider the following question: What is spiritual sexual health in recovery? Spiritual sexual health combines ethical behavior with internationally respected global agreements of sexual health. We will learn six fundamental principles of sexual health for all sexually active people. These principles are adapted from the World Health Organization and from the Religious Institute on Sexual Morality, Justice, and Healing (Haffner & Ott, 2005). The collective wisdom of these organizations will guide us to learn how recovery from drug addiction and alcoholism is an opportunity to develop fundamental spiritual and ethical principles of sexual health.

This lesson is not about religion and sex. Persons of all religious beliefs, creeds, and faiths (including those who are not religious) are welcome. Today's group will not discuss what your religion, faith, or sacred text says about sex. Some of you may believe in God; others may be uncertain about what you believe. Some of you may not believe in God. Believing in God is not necessary to develop spiritual or ethical principles of sexual health in recovery. Sexual health in recovery is about being aware of the relapse risk consequences of engaging in sexual behavior that conflicts with one's ethics and values. Women and men in recovery increase their likelihood of staying sober when they connect universal principles of sexual health with their personal spiritual and ethical values.

We will learn how practicing six fundamentals of sexual health can prevent random, impulsive, and poor sexual decisions that are often linked with drugs, alcohol, and sex. These six principles of sexual health provide a map to decrease fear of sexuality and relapse. We will use a deck of sex/drug-linked situation playing cards to learn each of these six principles of sexual health. Together we will practice applying each of them in a variety of sex/drug-linked situations. We will end this lesson by learning how to complete "The Sexuality and Spirituality in Recovery Inventory."

LECTURE

Leader: A central question for sexuality in recovery is: Why do I act against my better judgment when it comes to sex? When it comes to sex in recovery, why do I sometimes lose my will to maintain what some may call my moral compass? Researchers (Caron Treatment Centers, 2003; Reach, 2008) have been studying the various reasons for this human frailty among men and women addicted to drugs. They discovered that drug-dependent individuals discount and devalue the future consequences of their behavior more than nonaddicts do. It seems when the future looks empty and you do not know what tomorrow is going to look like that it is very likely that you will have insufficient willpower to listen to your better judgment.

Researcher Gerard Reach (Reach, 2008) provides an example of this concept. Consider accepting or refusing a cigarette.

Have two volunteers come to the front of the class. Have one offer the other a cigarette. Have the class discuss what immediate rewards the person might feel or desire as he or she decides whether or not to accept the cigarette.

Leader: What delayed rewards might the person desire? The moment of deciding whether or not to smoke requires a person to "decide between a large, but delayed reward (eg, health) and a small, but immediate reward (eg, smoking a cigarette)" (Reach, 2008, p. 7). The force of immediate desires compared with the long-term rewards depends on how long one must wait before the long-term reward.

Have the role-play participants discuss what long-term rewards might be worth the wait. Have them start with a reward as short as 1 minute or 5 minutes.

Leader: Dr. Reach proposes that the long term reward is not enough to explain why someone chooses to turn down the highly immediately rewarding choice to smoke. The long-term reward must be combined with a *recovery mental state*. A recovery mental state occurs when a person places a very high priority on the future that is much greater than the present. This is a skill that is learned and practiced in addiction treatment and recovery.

Remember, men and women who develop addictions tend not to excel in this area when compared to nonaddicts. Men and women in recovery may have remarkably high tendencies to focus on an immediate situation and give absolutely no priority to the future. A future 5 minutes, 5 hours, 5 days, 5 months, or 5 years from right now can easily be discounted. Devaluing and discounting the future is a fundamental process of drug dependence. Spirituality is a discipline for developing a belief in the future. Spirituality and sexual health is maintaining the willpower and discipline to believe in a future of sobriety and sexual health.

The fundamentals for sexual health are based on sexual health guidelines developed by the World Health Organization and The Religious Institute on Sexual Morality, Justice, and Healing. In 2002, the World Health Organization (we will call it the W-H-O) proposed a working definition of sexual health to include physical, emotional, mental, and social aspects of sexual life. They went on to expand sexual health as much more than just the absence of sexual diseases, dysfunctions, or medical illness. "Sexual health requires a positive and respectful approach to sexuality and sexual relationships, as well as the possibility of having pleasurable and safe sexual experiences, free of coercion, discrimination, and violence" (Coleman, 2007, p. 9).

We will see how several of these aspects of sexual health are integrated within the six principles of spiritual sexual health in recovery. Sexual health is more than a broad construction of internationally established minimum ground rules. Each person has a responsibility to know his or her own specific individual behaviors that characterize his or her vision of personal sexual health.

The "List of Life Behaviors of a Sexually Healthy Adult" (Lesson 6 appendix, C) was developed by experts in the United States and has been endorsed by other countries. It lists 30 behaviors that embody responsible and healthy adult sexual behavior. Several of these individual adult sexual health behaviors are directly relevant to recovery and prevention of relapse. The WHO report, the SIECUS List of Life Behaviors of a Sexually Healthy Adult (Coleman, 2007), and the

Religious Institute on Sexual Morality, Justice, and Healing state that healthy sexual relationships are the foundational principles within the six principles of sexual health in recovery.

Early recovery has some important dynamics that make these sexual health principles essential for discussing sex and sexuality in recovery. You may be interacting with a variety of people that are not usually part of your day-to-day life. Most of us have specific individual components of our sexual life that may not be the same as everyone else in this treatment program.

For example, you may be in a treatment program that involves a level of emotional closeness and intimacy that is very unfamiliar. Sometimes this closeness can become sexually stimulating. These principles can be very important in managing sexual feelings that arise out of the closeness and sharing among men and women in recovery. You may have left your home to be in a residential treatment setting to save your life, job, relationship, marriage, or to escape violence and danger. Adults living in a sober living home or residential treatment program have additional stressors of sharing rooms, living quarters, meals, and general living space with many other adults. This too can generate attractions, sexual feelings, and interests. These principles can assist with getting out of the immediate moments of sexual feelings and focusing on a bigger picture of recovery and prevention of a sex/drug-linked relapse.

Sexual health in recovery outlines six fundamentals of sexual health. These fundamentals provide a moral compass for creating your individual map for sexual health in recovery. Every person, from any culture, religion, or spiritual practice, can add to these values and principles in order to align with his or her religion, faith, or creedal belief system. The six fundamentals are a baseline for measuring sexual values and behavior in recovery. Aligning oneself with these six spiritual and ethical sexual health principles is a foundation for sexual health in recovery.

EXPERIENTIAL LEARNING

Leader: We are going to learn these principles one at a time. I have a deck of sex/drug-linked situation playing cards. On one side of each card is a brief description of a sexual situation. We will read the situation, discuss one of the principles, and then discuss how the principle will guide a person in recovery in resolving the situation. Let's start by reading a card from the deck.

Have a few cards that deal with the topic of consent preselected and put into a small deck. (See Lesson 6 appendix, A.) Have someone walk up to the front of the class and ask him or her to draw a card and read it out loud.

Leader: The first point on the moral compass is consent. Sexual health requires sex to be consensual. Consent means "voluntary cooperation" (Wertheimer, 2003, p. 124) and the go-ahead to try and reach sexual satisfaction and intimacy with willing partners (See Wertheimer, 2003, p. 125 for more discussion). Consent allows every woman and man to pursue a sexual life that is consistent with his or her sexual desires. Nonconsent forces an adult or child to have a sexual experience that he or she does not want or desire. Consent transforms the act of sex from an invasion, intrusion, or violation into an act of transformation. When I consent, I am saying, "I want this experience to have an effect on me, to change me, to give me something that I desire and I want you to provide it for me." How is consenting an issue in this sex/drug-linked situation?

Lead a discussion about consent. Reinforce key concepts such as voluntary cooperation, invasion, intrusion, violation, children/age of consent. Topics may include the following:

- *How drugs can be used to make someone incapable of giving consent (unconscious, in a blackout, or just not able to think or act to protect oneself).*
- *How being drunk or high is used as an explanation for engaging in forced or nonconsensual sex.*
- *How someone may assume that providing drugs means they are owed sex in return.*

Post a large compass titled "Sexual Health in Recovery" with six directions on the white board. As each new term is introduced, add it to a point on the compass. Begin by adding "consent" on the compass.

Leader: The second point on the moral compass is nonexploitive. Sexual health requires sex to be nonexploitive. Sexual health in recovery is not making use of somebody for sex unfairly. Exploitive sex is cruel, brutal, and oppressive. Exploitive sex deliberately causes pain and anguish by placing someone in a situation where choosing not to have sex may be more painful than choosing to have sex. Exploitive sex can be ruthless and insensitive to how the other person feels. Exploitive sex usually involves some form of harsh or cruel domination. Sex is nonexploitive when the person is old enough or mentally capable to use his or her cognitive and emotional capacities to make an informed decision. Sex is exploitive when intoxication is used as an excuse or permission to be exploitive.

Let's draw a card and discuss how the situation could be resolved without resorting to exploitation.

Have a few cards which deal with nonexploitation preselected and put into a small deck. (See Lesson 6 appendix, A.) Have someone walk up to the front of the class and ask him or her to draw a card and read it out loud.

Leader: How is nonexploitation an issue in this sex/drug-linked situation?

Lead a discussion. Reinforce key concepts such as being cruel, causing pain, placing someone in a situation to choose sex to avoid a more painful outcome, and being insensitive to how others feel. Exploitation is a fundamental behavior of an alcoholic or addict. Knowing when sexual behavior is exploitive will be a very important recovery tool. For many addicts, sexual exploitation was often a common means of having sex or providing sex to obtain drugs. The using world of addiction makes sexual exploitation a common element of the life of many addicts. The content of the stories may vary based on gender, age, and drug of choice. The common theme will be the role sex plays in gaining access to drugs, money, shelter, or a supplier. The painful consequences of the sex will often be overlooked for the immediate availability of drugs or of a sexual partner. It is important to emphasize the theme of the immediate reward system of addicts and their inability to focus on the longer term benefit of maintaining a sexual ethic or value.

Add "nonexploitive" to a point on the compass.

Leader: The third point on the moral compass is being protected from sexually transmitted infections (STIs) and unintended pregnancy. Sexual health in recovery requires that all partners are protected from STIs and unintended pregnancy. People are capable of protecting themselves and others from an STI and unintended pregnancy when they:

- Know their health status.
- Know if they have an STI.
- Get medical attention for treatment.
- Know how to manage a lifelong STI like herpes, hepatitis, or HIV.

- Know how to prevent pregnancy.
- Use contraception when desired.
- Take responsibility to prevent pregnancy.
- Not give full responsibility for contraception to their partner.
- "Seek further information about reproduction as needed" (Coleman, 2007, p. 11).

Leader: Let's draw a card and discuss how the situation could be resolved by protecting all partners from STIs and pregnancy.

Have a few cards that deal with the topic of protection from STIs and unintended pregnancy preselected and put into a small deck. (See Lesson 6 appendix, A.) Have someone walk up to the front of the class and ask him or her to draw a card and read it out loud.

Leader: How is protection from STIs and pregnancy an issue in this sex/drug-linked situation?

Lead a discussion. Reinforce key concepts: protection, knowledge of health status, medical treatment, protection against pregnancy, knowledge of contraception, taking responsibility. Discussion here may focus on how to know if you have an STI and how to negotiate protecting yourself from risk of STIs. Basic to sexual health in recovery is knowing your physical sexual health status. When was I last tested for all STIs? Is my current sexual behavior in recovery continuing to place me at risk for another STI? Do I know for certain if I am HIV negative or HIV positive? Not knowing one's HIV status is often more stressful than actually knowing a test result. Avoiding knowing HIV status can be a factor in relapse risk.

Add "protected from sexually transmitted infections and unintended pregnancy" to a point on the compass.

Leader: The fourth point on the moral compass is honesty. Sexual health in recovery requires that all partners present information and express themselves truthfully. Honest sex is direct and open with oneself and partners. It is candid and straightforward. Sexual health requires that the facts of what you say and do correspond with reality. Honesty creates a sexual relationship that deserves trust and makes you a person to be trusted. Honesty is sincere, accurate, and consistent with basic principles of recovery.

Let's draw a card and discuss how the situation could be resolved by honest communication.

Have a few cards that deal with the topic of honesty preselected and put into a small deck. (See Lesson 6 appendix, A.) Have someone walk up to the front of the class and ask him or her to draw a card and read it out loud.

Leader: How is honesty an issue in this sex/drug-linked situation?

Lead a discussion. Reinforce key concepts: truthful, direct, open, candid, straightforward, facts correspond with reality, trusted relationship, sincere, accurate, consistent with principles of recovery. Discussion points may center on when being honest is harmful to a relationship. What sexual information about my past is necessary to disclose in order to stay sober? With relapse prevention as the focus, the questions around disclosure are important to orient within basic sexual health safety. Honesty around an STI is essential for relapse prevention, as are honesty about contraception for prevention of pregnancy, honesty about not using drugs or alcohol (being abstinent), honesty about relationship status (e.g., I am married. I am in a committed monogamous relationship), honesty about needing to end an affair.
Add "honesty" to a point on the compass.

Leader: The fifth point on the moral compass is mutual pleasure. Sexual health in recovery is when each partner is interested in his or her partner's pleasure. Mutual pleasure is a giving and receiving of pleasure. Giving pleasure and receiving pleasure have different meanings for different people. These are some words that are associated with pleasure: both creating and expressing love, connection, attraction, caring, affection, helping someone achieve orgasm, allowing someone to help you achieve orgasm, having fun, enjoyment, play, stress relief.

These statements are from the *Declaration of Sexual Rights* endorsed by the World Congress on Sexology. "Sexual expression is more than erotic pleasure and sexual acts. Individuals have a right to express their sexuality through communication, touch, emotional expressions and love." "Sexual pleasure, including autoeroticism [masturbation], is a source of physical, psychological, intellectual and spiritual well being" (Coleman, 2007, p. 20).

Let's draw a card and discuss how the situation involves mutual pleasure.

Have a few cards that all deal with the topic of mutual pleasure preselected and put into a small deck. (See Lesson 6 appendix, A.) Have someone walk up to the front of the class and ask him or her to draw a card and read it out loud.

Leader: How is mutual pleasure an issue in this sex/drug-linked situation?

Lead a discussion. Reinforce key words: giving, receiving, helping and being helped to orgasm, enjoyment, play, stress relief, expression of love, connection, a right to which each participant has a claim. This area is addressed in several areas of the curriculum. Here the focus of discussion may be on how drugs or alcohol are used to decrease inhibitions for specific sex acts, either to give or receive. Participants may discuss the practice of using drugs in order to feel more romantic, more connected, or able to achieve orgasm. Some people may have used drugs to delay orgasm or to prolong the ability to have sex without having an orgasm.
Leader adds "mutual pleasure" to a point on the compass.

Leader: The last point on the moral compass is specific to sexual health in recovery. It is not directly from the WHO, SIECUS, or The Religious Institute. However, it is a basic sexual health boundary for all men and women addicted to drugs or alcohol. Sex in recovery must support a recovery program. Sex in recovery supports treatment goals and recovery goals. This is why it is so important to maintain a mental attitude about having a future. Without this mental attitude, it is very difficult to maintain the willpower to have a sexual life and a life in recovery.

Sexual health in recovery supports each person's individual recovery program from drug and alcohol addiction. Here are a few sexual health boundaries that support a recovery program:

- No drugs present
- No alcohol present
- No sexual partners under the influence of drugs/alcohol
- Partner negotiation of no drugs/alcohol prior to sexual relations
- Not being under the influence of drugs or alcohol
- No secrets from spouse, partner, children, recovery support network, sponsor, professional helpers, medical doctor

Leader: Let's draw a card and discuss how the situation involves supporting recovery.

Have a few cards that deal with the topic of supporting recovery preselected and put into a small deck. (See Lesson 6 appendix, A.) Have someone walk up to the front of the class and ask him or her to draw a card and read it out loud.

Leader: How is supporting recovery an issue in this sex/drug-linked situation?

Lead a discussion. Reinforce key words: no drugs or alcohol present during sex, no one under the influence of drugs or alcohol, sex that does not require secrets from your support system. A key relapse risk issue is sexual activity in recovery where the person in recovery is not using but the partner, spouse, dating partner, or casual sex partner has been drinking or using drugs. Often the attraction, desire, or interest in having sex can override better judgment about not combining sex with drugs or alcohol. Sexual intrigue within the recovery community can also be a significant relapse risk. Not wanting a sponsor to know about dating or having sex with someone in AA/NA can contribute greatly to relapse risk.
  Add "supports recovery program" to the final point on the compass.

TOPIC SKILL PRACTICE

Leader: Our last section for this class is to introduce you to a self-reflection tool you can use to think about sexuality and spirituality in recovery. "The Sexuality and Spirituality in Recovery Inventory" is a list of statements that reflect aspects of sexuality from a spiritual dimension. They describe sexuality and eroticism within a spiritual context. This is a tool you can use to initiate discussion with friends in recovery, lovers, sponsors, or with yourself during quiet reflection time. Filling out the inventory may provide you with motivation to learn more about sexuality and spirituality through books, religion, or spiritual leaders.

Leader passes around copies of the inventory (Lesson 6 appendix, B)

Let's read through each item together and give you a chance to think to yourself for moment about how you might answer the item. I won't ask you to share your answer. If you have any questions about what the item means, then circle "Not Sure." Remember, acknowledging what we do not know or are unsure about is a valuable tool in recovery.

Read each item, have a few moments to pause and reflect, and then proceed with the next item.

CLOSING

Leader: Now let's take a moment to bring the workshop to a close. Let's take a moment to again quiet ourselves, take a deep breath to quiet our minds, our hearts, and our spirits. In this quiet place, remind yourself how valuable it is to take the time to be honest, vulnerable, and committed to recovery. As you leave the group today, remind yourself that a satisfying sexual life is a vital and important part of recovery. The self-reflection and tools you learned today may become an important part of maintaining your recovery.

REFERENCES

Caron Treatment Centers. (2003). *Relapse and recovery: Behavioral strategies for change.* Wernersville, PA: Caron Treatment Centers.

Coleman, E. (2007). Creating a sexually healthy world through effective public policy. *International Journal of Sexual Health, 19*(3), 5–24.

de Chardin, P.T. (1970). *The essential teilhard—Selected passages from his works.* Retrieved March 1, 2009, from http://thinkexist.com/quotation/we_are_not_human_beings_having_a_spiritual/346797.html

Haffner, D., & Ott, K. (2005). *A time to speak: Faith communities and sexuality education* (2nd ed.). Norwalk, CT: Religious Institute on Sexual Morality, Justice, and Healing. Retrieved May 24, 2009, from www.religiousinstute.org/pubs/TimeToSpeak_07.pdf

Reach, G. (2008). A novel conceptual framework for understanding the mechanism of adherence to long term therapies. *Patient Preferences and Adherence, 2,* 7–19.

Wertheimer, A. (2003). *Consent to sexual relations.* Cambridge, UK: Cambridge University Press.

World Health Organization (WHO). (2006). *Defining sexual health: Report of a technical consultation on sexual health, 28–31 January 2002, Geneva.* Geneva, Switzerland: WHO Press.

LESSON 6 APPENDIX

A. Sex/Drug-Linked Circumstances

Here are some hypothetical sex/drug-linked circumstances. Make a copy of each situation and tape it to the back of a playing card. Make a deck with one situation on each card (Content of cards adapted from Wertheimer, 2003, pp. 277–286).

I encourage group leaders to write additional situations that may be specific to your treatment program, sexual concerns of your clients, or situations that you have encountered in your work with women and men in recovery. Have some blank cards on which you can do this. Be creative. Be specific. Use gender-neutral names; this will require participants to imagine the situations from various gender configurations. You may have discussions about how the situation is perceived differently when "Pat" and "Terry" are specifically male or female.

Exploitation

Abandonment: Pat and Terry drive in Pat's car to a secluded area. Terry resists Pat's offer of pot and sexual advances. Pat says, "Have sex with me or I will leave you here."

Exploitation

Crystal meth: Terry is Pat's connection for crystal. Terry tells Pat, "Have sex with me or I won't deliver the crystal." Pat cannot quickly find another connection.

Exploitation

Debt: Terry owes Pat $400. Terry says "Have sex with me as my payment, otherwise, I'm out of here."

Supporting Recovery

Liquid courage: Pat and Terry are dating. Terry is an alcoholic in recovery. Pat does not want to have intercourse until married. Pat feels guilty and ashamed of wanting to have intercourse. Pat gets drunk. After some kissing and fondling, Terry asks "Are you sure it's OK?" Pat lifts up her glass and says "Now it is!"

Consent

Force: Pat overpowers Terry physically, holds Terry down despite Terry's attempts to resist. Pat threatens Terry with more force if Terry continues to resist.

Honesty and Supporting Recovery

First high: Pat is an alcoholic. Pat has never used crystal. Terry offers Pat crystal at a party. Pat asks if this is really crystal. Terry says yes. Pat gets really high for the first time. Terry suggests they go home together. Pat agrees.

Consent

Guilt: Terry wants to have intercourse with Pat. Pat has no idea that Terry wants intercourse. Terry has also told Pat that Terry will not have intercourse in the first year of sobriety. Terry feels guilty about asking for intercourse with Pat because Terry wants to be celibate in the first year of recovery. Pat and Terry get high. While Terry is saying "No, please don't," Pat holds Terry down and penetrates Terry.

Consent

Pat does not know Terry. Terry does not know Pat. They ride the same subway to work each day. Pat moves next to Terry when the subway is very crowded. Pat touches Terry between the legs and acts like nothing is happening. Terry says nothing. Pat gets off the subway at the next stop.

Protected from STIs and HIV

Dishonesty

HIV: Terry makes advances toward Pat. Terry knows Pat shoots crystal. Terry asks Pat, "Have you been tested for HIV?" Pat tested negative 6 months ago, but tested positive last month. Pat says, "I tested negative 6 months ago."

Protected from STIs and HIV

Dishonesty

HIV: Terry makes advances toward Pat. Terry knows Pat shoots crystal. Terry asks Pat, "Have you been tested for HIV?" Pat tested HIV positive 6 months ago. Pat says, "I tested negative six months ago, I'm clean."

Dishonesty

Apathetic boundaries: Pat and Terry meet in a bar. Pat does not care about a new partner's marital or relationship status. After many drinks, Pat asks Terry, "Are you married?" Terry thinks a truthful answer will stop Pat from wanting to have sex. Terry lies. Pat believes Terry.

Supporting Recovery

New Year's Eve: Pat and Terry are a couple. They get very drunk at a New Year's Eve party. They take a taxi home. They stagger into their house and have sex.

Protected from STIs and HIV

Dishonesty

HIV nondisclosure: Terry makes sexual advances towards Pat. Terry has a "if I am not asked I do not disclose or talk about being positive" policy. Pat does not ask. Terry does not disclose.

Supporting Recovery

Inhibitions: When Pat has a few drinks Pat is less inhibited. Pat is currently dating Terry. Pat told Terry, "I am not ready for sex yet." Pat and Terry go out for dinner and Pat drinks an entire bottle of wine. When Terry suggests they go home and have sex, Pat says, "Why not?"

Exploitation

Homeless risk: Pat rents a room from Terry. Pat is several months behind in paying rent. Terry knows Pat is a drug addict. Terry says, "If you have sex with me once a week until you pay your rent I won't evict you."

Mutual Pleasure

Caring: Pat and Terry have been married for many years. Pat finds much fulfillment in being a spouse and parent. Pat's interests revolve around the family's interests. Pat maintains an active sexual relationship with Terry. Pat is emotionally fulfilled by this relationship but does not experience the same level of erotic pleasure as Terry.

Consent

Children: Pat and Terry are in the first grade and are neighbors. Pat and Terry are playing together in Terry's house. Terry is interested in seeing what Pat's genitals looks like. Pat is interested in showing Terry. They start to play doctor and end up with their clothes off, looking at each others' bodies.

Consent
Mutual Pleasure

Friends: Pat and Terry are both in their early 20s; both are friends and are single. Both talk about how lonely they are and complain about not having anyone to date. They both like each other. Terry proposes that they have sex.

Honest
Mutual Pleasure

Love: Pat and Terry are a long-term couple. Pat proposes that they have sex. Terry is not in the mood. Terry is concerned how long it has been since they have made love. Terry feels much closer to Pat when they are having regular enjoyable sex. Terry wants to show Pat "that I really love you" and Terry agrees to have sex.

Protected From Pregnancy

Ovulation: Pat and Terry are trying to conceive a child. Terry monitors when ovulation is most likely to occur. Both Terry and Pat know that the best time for conception is right when the egg is released from the ovaries or one or two days before ovulation. Terry says, "This is the right time." Pat and Terry have intercourse.

Honest
Mutual Pleasure

Smile: Pat and Terry have been dating. They have not had intercourse. Terry proposes that they go back to Pat's apartment. Pat agrees. When they enter the apartment, Terry kisses Pat. Terry points to Pat's bedroom and says, "How about we go in there?" Pat smiles and follows Terry into the bedroom, not saying another word.

Mutual Pleasure

Sweethearts: Terry and Pat are both 14. They are in ninth grade at the same high school. They have been dating since the beginning of the school year. They have sex several times a week.

Consent

Facebook: Terry and Pat are friends in the same Facebook network. Terry has a thing for (is attracted to and interested in) Pat. Terry writes to Pat and the entire conversation can be read by everyone on "Wall to Wall" (conversation script can be read by anyone in their network). Pat is uncomfortable with Terry talking about this attraction in Facebook rather than in person. Pat is not sure what to say.

B. The Sexuality and Spirituality in Recovery Inventory

Rate yourself on each item. Each item is an opportunity to reflect and measure your current sexual behavior as it relates to the six foundations of sexual health in recovery

First measure how you are doing on the six fundamentals (rate yourself based on your sexual life since you last filled out this questionnaire. If this is your first time filling it out, rate yourself based on your sexual life since you became sober.

Read each item, think about each item, and take your time. Reflect on how much you agree with each statement.

FIRST REFLECT ON THE SIX FUNDAMENTAL ETHICAL AND SPIRITUAL PRINCIPLES

	STRONGLY DISAGREE	DISAGREE	AGREE	STRONGLY AGREE	
1. The physical act of sex has always been consensual.	1	2	3	4	Not sure
2. I have not engaged in sex with someone as a result of exploiting them (or being exploited).	1	2	3	4	Not sure
3. I have protected myself and my partners from sexually transmitted infections (and pregnancy, if desired).	1	2	3	4	Not sure
4. I have been honest with my sexual partners.	1	2	3	4	Not sure
5. I have been focused on my partner's and my own sexual pleasure.					
6. I am supporting my goals for recovery in my sexuality.	1	2	3	4	Not sure

WHEN I REFLECT ON MY SEXUAL ETHICS AND SPIRITUALITY TODAY

	STRONGLY DISAGREE	DISAGREE	AGREE	STRONGLY AGREE	
1. The physical act of sex in not always my ultimate goal.	1	2	3	4	Not sure
2. Sex is an important component of how I express my whole being.	1	2	3	4	Not sure
3. I ask for what I need in my sexual relationships.	1	2	3	4	Not sure
4. I want to build a committed sexual relationship with someone I love.	1	2	3	4	Not sure
5. A sexual experience with my intimate partner can be a way to touch each other's souls.	1	2	3	4	Not sure
6. I like to lose myself and meld with my partner during sex as if the boundary of skin-to-skin contact is lost and a sense of timelessness exists.	1	2	3	4	Not sure
7. Sexual pleasure is a haven for me where I feel free to express myself.	1	2	3	4	Not sure
8. I find a powerful pleasure in hidden, mysterious, and suggestive erotic activity.	1	2	3	4	Not sure
9. My body's erotic nature is a virtue.	1	2	3	4	Not sure

WHEN I REFLECT ON MY SEXUAL ETHICS AND SPIRITUALITY TODAY (CONTINUED)

	STRONGLY DISAGREE	DISAGREE	AGREE	STRONGLY AGREE	
10. I like to abandon myself to my senses during sex and give up my need to understand everything that is happening.	1	2	3	4	Not sure
11. Sex and sexuality can be a mystical experience.	1	2	3	4	Not sure
12. My body and the sensations my body brings me can serve my spiritual goals.	1	2	3	4	Not sure
13. Everything I do, everything I contact, every event in life, has spiritual significance.	1	2	3	4	Not sure
14. Sex is an opportunity to leave ordinary reality behind by entering deeply into sensation, imagination, and passion.	1	2	3	4	Not sure
15. Part of my spiritual practice is to cultivate affection and sensuality.	1	2	3	4	Not sure
16. My spirituality is partly defined by whom I love.	1	2	3	4	Not sure
17. My sexuality is something I make through my everyday experimentation with sensation, sex, and pleasure.	1	2	3	4	Not sure

(continued)

WHEN I REFLECT ON MY SEXUAL ETHICS AND SPIRITUALITY TODAY (CONTINUED)

	STRONGLY DISAGREE	DISAGREE	AGREE	STRONGLY AGREE	
18. I can use prayer and conscious contact with my Higher Power to develop my spiritual sexual life.	1	2	3	4	Not sure
19. I use my spiritual life to support me in being honest, vulnerable, and open with my sexuality.	1	2	3	4	Not sure
20. My spirituality depends on me fully embracing my sexuality.	1	2	3	4	Not sure

From *A Time to Speak: Faith Communities and Sexuality Education* (2nd ed.), by D. Haffner & K. Ott, 2005. Norwalk, CT: Religious Institute on Sexual Morality, Justice, and Healing. Retrieved May 24, 2009, from www.religiousinstute.org/pubs/TimeToSpeak_07.pdf

C. List of Life Behaviors of a Sexually Healthy Adult

- Appreciate one's own body.
- Seek further information about reproduction as needed.
- Affirm that human development includes sexual development, which may or may not include reproductive or sexual experience.
- Interact with all genders in respectful and appropriate ways.
- Affirm one's own sexual orientation and respect the sexual orientations of others.
- Express love and intimacy in appropriate ways.
- Develop and maintain meaningful relationships.
- Avoid exploitive or manipulative relationships.
- Make informed choices about family options and relationships.
- Exhibit skills that enhance personal relationships.
- Identify and live according to one's own values.
- Take responsibility for one's own behavior.
- Practice effective decision making.
- Communicate effectively with family, peers, and romantic partners.
- Enjoy and express one's sexuality throughout life.
- Express one's sexuality in ways that are congruent with one's values.
- Discriminate between life-enhancing sexual behaviors and those that are harmful to self and/or others.
- Express one's sexuality while respecting the rights of others.
- Seek new information to enhance one's sexuality.
- Use contraception effectively to avoid unintended pregnancy.
- Prevent sexual abuse.
- Seek early prenatal care.
- Avoid contracting or transmitting a sexually transmitted infection, including HIV.
- Practice health-promoting behaviors, such as regular check-ups, breast and testicular self-exams, and early identification of potential problems.
- Demonstrate tolerance for people with different sexual values and lifestyles.
- Exercise democratic responsibility to influence legislation dealing with sexual issues.
- Assess the impact of family, cultural, religious, media, and societal messages on one's thoughts, feelings, values, and behaviors related to sexuality.

- Promote the rights of all people to accurate sexuality information.
- Avoid behaviors that exhibit prejudice and bigotry.
- Reject stereotypes about the sexuality of diverse populations (Coleman, 2007, p. 11).

Sexual Past

7 Sexual Development

CORE CONCEPT

Recovery is a process that involves looking back at life as part of going forward in sobriety. Men and women's sexual history and development is an important component of looking back. The process of looking back at our sexual development often creates feelings of both excitement and fear. The way addicts will come to better understand their current sexual feelings and actions must include an honest and open look at their sexual past. However, a strong motivation to recover may run directly into an equally strong fear of discussing our sexual past. When addicts in recovery develop a deeper understanding and acceptance of their sexual past, they increase the likelihood of remaining sober.

The purpose of this session is to learn a skill related to understanding our sexual past. It is not a group designed to process each participant's feelings and thoughts about his or her personal sexual history. The majority of the session will be spent looking at common sexual development milestones and their possible link with drugs and alcohol. We will focus on valuing ambivalent feelings and taking the time to consider sexual choices in recovery that may have a history of being linked with getting high or drinking. Participants will practice using the "Looking Back/Looking Forward Exercise" to evaluate their feelings of sexual uncertainty or indecision in recovery.

BELIEF STATEMENT

Sexual health in recovery is the ability to increase awareness about the role of drugs and alcohol in sexual development.

OBJECTIVES

Participants will
- Identify events and issues that mark sexual development.
- Discuss connection between sexual development and drug and alcohol use history.
- Practice using the "Looking Back/Looking Forward Exercise" for analyzing ambivalence about sexual choices in recovery.

CHANGE GOALS

- Increase knowledge about stages of sexual development.
- Increase knowledge of drug and alcohol use/abuse in sexual developmental history.
- Clarify feelings and thoughts about role of drugs and alcohol in sexual development.

REQUIRED READING FOR GROUP LEADER

- *Sex Matters for Women: A Complete Guide to Taking Care of Your Sexual Self* (Foley, Kope & Sugrue, 2002) is a comprehensive guide to women's sexual health. It is resolute in advocating for women to know their sexual story and its role in shaping sexual attitudes, inhibitions, and negative influences. Many chapters in this book will be mentioned as required reading for leading this curriculum. Chapters 1 and 2 focus on sexual development from birth to old age. Understanding key developmental milestones in sexual development separate from the sex/drug link will be important for leading the group as they process writing their "Sexual Development Life Cycle Time Line."

- The Sexuality Information and Education Council of the United States' (SIECUS) *Guidelines for Comprehensive Sexuality Education: Kindergarten–12th Grade* (SIECUS, 2004) is a good source of sexual development milestones presented in a format for teaching at various age levels. The first key concept in this curriculum (pp. 24–32) is human development. Each developmental stage outlines sexual health–based developmental messages. These messages are excellent examples of sex-positive language and tone for discussing sexual development. Group leaders can refer to this document to become more familiar with easy-to-state sentences about sexual development.
- *Men's Sexual Health: Fitness for Satisfying Sex* (McCarthy & Metz, 2007) is a reference book for male sexual health and development that I recommend having for source material in leading this curriculum. Chapter 3, "Boys to Men: What Is Normal and Healthy?" provides an excellent overview of male developmental milestones as preparation for this lesson. The tone of the book makes for an excellent resource for clients and residents, especially for men who may prefer reading information privately before discussion.

RECOMMENDED MATERIALS FOR GROUP LEADER

- John Money's *Principles of Developmental Sexology* (1999) is the first book to devise an original system of developmental categories and stages for sexual development that is vigilant in using science, data, and empirical evidence to construct a comprehensive theory of child and adolescent sexual development and maturation. This book is for the trainer who aspires to develop a sound basis in sexological training as a foundation for teaching this course. Read it slowly. Money's writing is dense and must be read with concentration. He was a big thinker. This book is the summation of his life's work (he died in 2006) and is an original work of sexual science that is the foundation for how many sexual health experts think about a variety of sexual problems and disorders.
- The Magnus Hirschfeld Archive for Sexology is the "world's largest web site on human sexuality" (Haeberle, 2008). The mission of the Hirschfeld Archive is to "preserve and protect sexual

health through original research and by collecting, analyzing, and disseminating scientific information from other sources" (Haeberle, 2008). Offering content in 11 different languages, the archive provides sexual health information for non-English speakers or clients for whom English is a second language. It has excellent resource material on basic sexual development and is another good source for clients in treatment who want professional online sexual health information (the archive is available at http://www.2hu-berlin.de/sexology/index.htm).

REQUIRED MATERIALS FOR THE LESSON

- An mp3 player and music selection
- Blackboard, white board, or flip chart
- The "Sexual Development Life Cycle Time Line" sheets (one copy for each participant) (Lesson 7 appendix, A)
- "Looking Back/Looking Forward Exercise" (one copy for each participant) (Lesson 7 appendix, B)

OPENING

Opening Music: *Have quiet music playing as participants enter the room and ready themselves (optional).*

Leader: As we sit quietly and focus on being here, let us clear our minds of where we have been and focus on being in this moment.

Opening Poem/Reading:

Our present sexual feelings and actions do not exist in a vacuum. They are molded and influenced by everything that has happened to us in the past. By working with our past and honestly naming all that has happened to us—our sexual training within our families, our childhood experiences, our adolescent sexual experiences, our choice of partners, our sexual behavior while drinking or using drugs—we can move into a new level of sexual freedom and expansion. When this happens, our sexual feelings and actions will have to do with today, not with some unknown carryover from yesterday.

—S. Covington, *Awakening Your Sexuality* (1991)

GROUP INTRODUCTION

Have a group member volunteer to read aloud.

Welcome to the sexual health in recovery group. We are here to talk about sex and how our sexual lives affect recovery from drug and alcohol addiction. Some people in recovery risk a relapse because of their sexual behavior at the treatment center or away from the treatment program. This is a place to talk about sexual behavior and sexual health so we can be abstinent from drugs and alcohol. It is also a place to learn about sexual behavior and situations that put men and women in recovery at risk for not completing this treatment program.

Sexual health in recovery is a time to talk about human sexuality and sexual health in a respectful and informed manner. We encourage everyone to be as honest and open as you can be. You are not required to reveal anything about your current or past sexual behavior that would be uncomfortable to discuss. It is important to listen to each other. For some of us, our sexual behavior is the most serious risk to staying in recovery. For others, our sexual behavior gets us into dangerous situations that are triggers to use or drink. A few of us may have little concern about how our sexual behavior contributes to relapse. This group is an opportunity for everyone to learn about the important connection between recovery and sexual health.

LESSON INTRODUCTION

Ask another group member to volunteer to read aloud.

The purpose of today's sexual health in recovery group is to discuss how drugs and alcohol influence our sexual history and development. We believe that women and men in recovery will increase their likelihood of staying sober when they increase their awareness about the role of drugs and alcohol in their sexual development. Most of what we have learned about sex has come about by trial and error, blunders and successes. Most women and men in treatment have made serious sexual missteps when under the influence of drugs and alcohol. Talking about our sexual development in relation to our use of drugs and alcohol can reveal how our current patterns of sexual behavior may increase our risk of relapse. This self-knowledge will help us stay sober.

After a brief beginning that will teach us about boundaries, we will divide into groups for men and women. Each group will brainstorm a list of important events in human sexual development. We will compare our list with what the experts have to say about significant sexual developmental milestones. We will learn how to fill out a sexual time line and complete our own personal sexual developmental time line. We will highlight specific stages in our own sexual development linked with drug and alcohol use. We will practice an exercise that looks back on a sex/drug-linked sexual experience and then looks forward by imagining the sex in recovery options/choices for you now.

LECTURE

Leader: Today we are going to talk about sexual development. It may sound pretty straightforward and not too complicated. But I think we will find putting our ideas about sexual development into words is not always so easy. We may need to talk about things we are not used to talking about in groups. We may be unsure if something in our own sexual development is typical or unusual. Almost everyone wants his or her own sexual development to be normal.

Today we will discuss sexual development from the perspective of the kinds of events, behaviors, actions, body changes, and sexual choices that occur as we grow from infancy to adulthood. A goal for today is to listen to what others have to say. We may find some reassurance in hearing that someone else experienced events similar to our own sexual development. Because the experience of sexual development is central to whether it is experienced as a girl or a boy we are going to separate into two groups for the remainder of the session.

Leader: Before we separate into our two groups, we want to do a brief discussion about boundaries. I know we hear a lot of talk about healthy and unhealthy boundaries for people in recovery. We need to talk for a few minutes about unhealthy boundaries for when we break into two groups in the sexual behavior relapse prevention group. When we meet together as an entire group, the boundaries are different because we all share the same experience together. If someone shares some personal information in the group, it is not private from other members of the group. We all heard it together. When we break into separate groups, the boundary around privacy is different. What the women share in their group and what the men share in their group is not to be shared by you with the members of the other group. You are free to share whatever you want about yourself and what you shared in the separate group. But it is important to respect the privacy and emotional boundaries of the other group members by not disclosing their personal information with persons who were not in the group.

Separate the group into two groups, men and women, for the remainder of the session. From this point forward the groups should convene in separate rooms, and each group is facilitated by one (or two) group leader(s). The lesson plans are identical for both groups, other than a change in pronouns. (Note: Transgender men or women or intersex clients will decide which group based upon gender assignment or identity when children and adolescents)

Leader: We are going to start by listing significant events in a person's sexual development. We are going to make a list of important sexual life cycle changes, events, and developments that are typical for men/women. We want to make sure our list includes physical body changes, sex acts, discovering of sexual orientation, harmful or traumatic sexual events, as well as falling in love and developing meaningful love relationships. We are not going to put them in any particular order. We will worry about that later. The one distinction we will make is that we will write sexual developments that are under our control in black and will mark the ones that are not under our control in red.

Begin taking examples from the group. Encourage participants to be specific, use clear and respectful language. Give everyone a chance to contribute. Do not worry about editing or organizing the examples in any order. Consider asking participants to add the following events if they have not already done so:

- *Physical body maturation,*
- *Genital maturation,*
- *Begin having sexual fantasies,*
- *First crush,*
- *First love,*
- *Begin to masturbate,*
- *Emotional sexual abuse,*
- *Physical sexual abuse,*
- *Sexual health problems,*
- *HIV concerns begin,*
- *First experimentation with same-sex sexual behavior,*
- *First sexual intercourse,*
- *First long-term relationship,*
- *Pregnancy (planned or unplanned),*

- *Termination of pregnancy,*
- *Marriage,*
- *Developing sexual identity other than exclusively heterosexual,*
- *Identify as lesbian, gay, bisexual, transgender, and*
- *Develop positive sense of sexual orientation.*

Leader: You all did a great job. It is not often that we talk in groups saying all the sexual words and content that we just did. Let's take just a minute or two and talk about how we are all feeling right now.

Allow time for discussion.

EXPERIENTIAL LEARNING

Leader: We are now going to turn our attention to writing our own personal sexual life cycle time line. The time line has two important components.

Leader draws a sample time line on the wall. (See Lesson 7 appendix, A.)

Leader: On the line going left to right, we have the years of life divided into increments of 5 years starting with birth. Along the side of the timeline we have a rating scale of plus 10 to minus 10 with the zero point intersecting with the time line. For each significant event in your sexual development time line I want to you rate how painful or pleasurable the event was. The plus side is pleasurable and the minus side is painful. So if you started masturbating when you were 12 and it was a pretty pleasurable experience, you might mark it like this.

Show example by placing the mark on the timeline, writing next to the mark what the event was.

Leader: Are there any questions about how to do this? OK, I will now hand out a blank sexual life cycle sheet to you that you can fill out about yourself in today's group. We will take time to quietly fill these out and begin to get a sense of the important, meaningful, pleasurable, and painful aspects of our sexual development.

Hand out the "Sexual Life Cycle Time Line" sheets. Allow participants a chance to fill them out.

Leader: Now, let's return to the group list of sexual developmental events. Which sexual developmental stages typically involve use or abuse of drugs/alcohol? Let's circle any of the events we have on our general sexual development list that may be linked with using drugs or alcohol.

Participants volunteer their opinions; consider all suggestions given and continue to circle items on the list until group is done.

Leader: Let's return one last time to our personal sexual time lines and circle the events that included drugs or alcohol. This can be an effective way to visually see the association between your sexual development and how it may have been affected by drugs and alcohol. So now we will take a few moments and complete your time lines with the circles around the events that included drug and alcohol use. We will talk together about this exercise in a few minutes.

Give group a few minutes to complete task. There may be questions or discussion. Ask the group to do this part quietly and with themselves.

Leader: OK, now let's make our own list of the sexual developmental events that you circled on your lists. If you do not want to volunteer this information, it is OK. Let's make a list of sexual developmental events that people have experienced when high or drunk.

Make a list on the board. Ask group members to describe which drug was used with each developmental event. See if some members of the group were under the influence for the same developmental event but used a different drug. The differences are interesting. Point out to the group how the same sexual developmental event was approached differently by different group members.

TOPIC SKILL PRACTICE

Leader: We found that some of you in the group approached the same sexual developmental milestone differently. This is important to remember. There is never just one way to approach new, different, or stressful sexual situations. In recovery we are always looking at ways to solve a situation without choosing to use drugs or alcohol. When it comes to sexual situations, this is not always an easy choice. Sometimes the sexual situation seems impossible to approach without drugs. Sometimes we think we will only enjoy a particular sexual situation if we have used.

This may lead to uncertain or unclear choices. We may think it is not possible to be sexual without using. This is an important time to stop and assess our undecided feelings and thoughts.

Researchers who have studied how people change have found that wanting to change and *not* wanting to change all at the same time is a normal and important part of moving toward change. This feeling is called ambivalence. Feeling ambivalent about sexual desires and behavior is a difficult feeling for people in early recovery. We are going to teach you a recovery tool you can use when you are really ambivalent about a sexual situation that is a risk for drug or alcohol use.

Hand out "Looking Back/Looking Forward Exercise" (Lesson 7 appendix, B).

Leader: This exercise can be used when you are feeling conflicted or uncertain about whether to do a particular sexual behavior. Feeling undecided and uncertain about sexual choices and options is going to happen for all of us from time to time. It will happen more frequently in early recovery. This exercise is a tool to assist you in exploring your ambivalent feelings. By looking back and looking forward, sometimes we do a better job of resolving a present conflict within ourselves. We will practice using this recovery tool.

Ask a group member to describe a sexual situation in early recovery that many people feel conflicted, uncertain, or ambivalent about. Situations offered by group members may include:

- *Getting emotionally involved with someone and feeling rejected if he or she doesn't feel the same about me,*
- *Having sex sober,*
- *Not wanting to take antidepressants because of the sexual side effects,*
- *Being OK with having sex,*
- *Feeling worried because I am so anxious because I do not know if I can be sexual,*
- *Feeling that raw sex is no longer an option,*
- *Feeling that being sexually excited will trigger using memories, and*
- *Thinking that being single means getting high.*

Write the situation on the board. Go through each item in the "Looking Back/Looking Forward Exercise." Fill in each item as someone would who is answering the questions for themselves. After completing the exercise on both sides, ask the group if they understand or see anything differently after the exercise. Invite participants to discuss any perception changes, thought changes, or different options they had not thought of before doing the exercise. Ambivalence may remain, but are there any additional compelling motivations for approaching this sexual situation without getting high?

Leader: Before we end our group today, let's take a few minutes to individually fill out the "Looking Back/Looking Forward Exercise." You can use your sexual time lines to help you remember or have greater clarity about your sexual past, to clarify the benefits and drawbacks of the behavior. Notice what you rated highly on your pleasure scale on your time line. Notice what you rated highly on your pain scale on your time line. Now take a few minutes to fill out this worksheet by considering a specific sexual behavior or action that you are currently feeling ambivalent about. If you do not currently have an ambivalent situation, predict a future sexual situation that you imagine will generate ambivalent feelings. This sheet is just for you, and we will not ask you to share it with the group today. Some of you may want to talk with your sponsor, a counselor, or some one you trust as a result of filling this sheet out.

CLOSING

Leader: Now let's take a moment to bring the workshop to a close. Let's take a moment to again quiet ourselves, take a deep breath to quiet our minds, our hearts, and our spirit. In this quiet place, remind yourself how valuable it is to take the time to be honest, vulnerable, and committed to recovery. As you leave the group today, remind yourself that a satisfying sexual life is a vital and important part of recovery. The self-reflection and tools you learned today may become an important part of maintaining your recovery.

REFERENCES

Covington, S. (1991). *Awakening your sexuality: A guide for recovering women.* Center City, MN: Hazelden.

Foley, S., Kope, S., & Sugrue, D. (2002). *Sex matters for women: A complete guide to taking care of your sexual self.* New York: The Guilford Press.

Haeberle, E. (2008). Magnus Hirschfeld Archive for Sexology. Retrieved from http://www2.hu-berlin.de/sexology/

McCarthy, B., & Metz, M. (2007). *Men's sexual health: Fitness for satisfying sex.* Boca Raton, FL: CRC Press.

Money, J. (1999). *Principles of developmental sexology.* New York: Continuum Publishing Company.

Sexuality Information and Education Council of the United States. (2004). *Guidelines for comprehensive sexuality education: Kindergarten–12th grade.* Retrieved March 1, 2009, from SIECUS.org_data/global/images/guidelines.pdf

LESSON 7 APPENDIX

A. Sexual Development Life Cycle Time Line

The "Sexual Development Life Cycle Time Line" is adapted from Covington's "Sexual/Chemical Lifeline" (1991, p. 118).

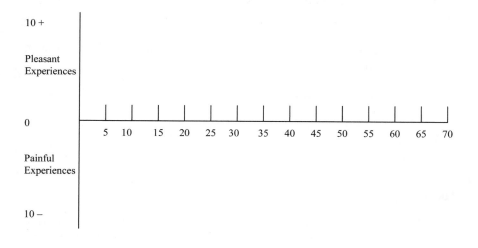

B. Looking Back/Looking Forward Exercise

This exercise can be used when you are feeling of two minds about a particular sexual behavior. Feeling undecided and uncertain about sexual choices and options is going to happen for all of us from time to time. It will happen more frequently in early recovery. This exercise is a tool to assist you in exploring your ambivalent feelings. By looking back and looking forward, sometimes we do a better job of resolving a present conflict within ourselves.

I feel uncertain and undecided about the following sexual choice, behavior, or desire.

_____

_____

_____

Looking Back

Describe a time in your sexual development before you ever used drugs or alcohol when you engaged in the sexual behavior that you are currently feeling ambivalent about.

_____

_____

_____

If you have never engaged in this behavior without using drugs or alcohol, describe what you remember about the first time you engaged in this behavior.

_____

_____

_____

_____

How did the presence of drugs help or hurt your first time with this particular sexual experience?

_____

_____

_____

Looking Forward

Describe the choices you would like to make in recovery regarding this particular sexual behavior.

_____

_____

_____

If you have never engaged in this behavior without using drugs or alcohol, describe what you think will be the benefits of being sober during the sexual experience.

_____

_____

_____

_____

If you have never engaged in this behavior without using drugs or alcohol, describe what you think will be the fears and drawbacks of being sober during the sexual experience.

_____

_____

_____

_____

The choice I can consider making today about this sexual behavior that will increase the likelihood of staying sober is:

_____

_____

_____

_____

_____

You can use this worksheet any time you are confronted with a difficult sexual choice. By remembering your past and looking at your hope for the future, you may get clearer about resolving your uncertainty.

8

Nonconsensual Sex

CORE CONCEPT

Experts now recognize childhood sexual abuse as a risk factor in all forms of drug dependence (Rosellini, 2002). "At least two-thirds of patients in drug abuse treatment centers say they were physically or sexually abused as children" (Swan, 1998). Women who experience any type of sexual abuse or nonconsensual sex in childhood may be three times more likely than unabused girls to report drug dependence as adults (Kendler et al., 2000). Researchers from the Harvard Medical School and McLean Hospital found that repeated sexual abuse during childhood causes physical changes in the brain that can explain why abused children often develop substance abuse problems (Anderson, Teicher, Polcari, & Renshaw, 2002).

Nonconsensual sexual relations are a violation of bodily integrity and sexual self-rule and control. This leads to harmful distress and psychological injury. Some sexual abuse survivors may themselves commit forced sexual violence/rape or use drugs to manipulate another adult or child into sex. Sobriety may lead to an increase in thinking about or remembering sexual abuse or committing sexual violence.

Participants will learn important information about sexual abuse and drug addiction/alcoholism. Most of the session will divide into two groups: one for men and the other women. Each group will discuss gender differences in experiencing and responding to sexual abuse. Everyone will learn and practice the "Self-Soothing Checklist" to regulate emotional states resulting from thoughts and memories of sexual abuse.

BELIEF STATEMENT

Sexual health in recovery is the ability to manage feelings linked with history of nonconsensual sex.

OBJECTIVES

Participants will
- Define sexual abuse and discuss common and differing consequences for male and female survivors.
- Learn to incorporate physical relaxation exercises in response to feelings associated with sexual abuse.
- Practice using the "Self-Soothing Checklist."
- Integrate use of the "Self-Soothing Checklist" for increasing internal safety when aware of feelings and symptoms connected with sexual abuse.

CHANGE GOALS

- Challenge myths and misinformation about frequency and consequences of sexual abuse and other forms of nonconsensual sex.
- Identify common thoughts, feelings, and relationship issues for men and women with a history of traumatic nonconsensual sex.
- Manage feelings and emotions that may arise in anticipation of discussing or remembering sexual abuse as the first skill in addressing sexual abuse as part of recovery.

REQUIRED READING FOR GROUP LEADER

Men and women in treatment are likely to have experienced sexual abuse. A smaller percentage may have committed rape or nonconsensual or exploitive sex. Two chapters from *Consent to Sexual Relations* (Wertheimer, 2003) are essential for conducting this workshop. Chapter 4, "The Psychology of Perpetrators," addresses the psychology of forced nonconsensual sex (Wertheimer, 2003, pp. 70–88). Work with sexual abuse survivors is greatly improved when a counselor has a working understanding of the motives and basis for men (and a much lower frequency for women) who rape. Chapter 6, "The Value of Consent," reviews the multifaceted and intricate necessity for men and women to "seek emotional intimacy and sexual fulfillment with willing partners" (Wertheimer, 2003, p. 125).

RECOMMENDED MATERIALS FOR GROUP LEADER

- *Beginning to Heal* by Ellen Bass and Laura Davis (1993). Although not a recent publication, it is written in a straightforward manner, making for an easy-to-read resource for leaders and clients alike. The book outlines stages of recovery from sexual abuse for women. The authors' model for healing is readily transferable within drug and alcohol recovery.
- *Victims No Longer* by Mike Lew (1989) is a standard resource for men beginning to explore childhood or adolescent sexual abuse. This is an excellent resource for facilitators who will lead the men's breakout group session. Contains many first-person accounts of men in recovery from sexual abuse.
- Personal Life Media (PersonalLifeMedia.com) is a Web site that offers talk shows, reality audio, interviews, tips, guided exercises, and frank discussion delivered via streams, podcasts, and blogs. In "Sex Love and Intimacy: Episode 27," Wendy Maltz, an internationally known sex educator and therapist, discusses healing sexuality with host Chip August (*Wendy Maltz: Healing our Sexuality*, 2009). This 30-minute interview is a good example of an expert sex therapist and author discussing sexual trauma and addressing the effects of sexual trauma on sexual health. The interview explores the differences between obligation and choice, shame and self-esteem, power and empowerment, having sex and making authentic love. Maltz describes a path from sexual abuse survivor to having a fulfilling sex life.
- Encyclopedia of Mental Disorders (http://www.minddisorders. com/) is a Web-based listing of over 150 mental disorders. From

the home page, search for "anxiety reduction techniques." This is excellent source material for understanding the physiological basis for the self-soothing exercises.

- EQI.org is Web page written by international traveler and peace activist Steve Hein (2009). It contains information about emotional intelligence. The *Feeling Words* list contains over 3,000 words. It is an excellent resource for Spanish-language feeling words.

REQUIRED MATERIALS FOR THE LESSON

- An mp3 player and music selection
- Computer and projection screen for opening poem/reading
- Blackboard, white board, or flip chart
- "Self-Soothing Checklist" worksheet (one copy for each participant) (Lesson 8 appendix, A)
- "Sexual Trauma Resource List" (one copy for each participant) (Lesson 8 appendix, B)
- 3 × 5 index cards

OPENING

Opening Music: *Have quiet music playing as participants enter the room and ready themselves (optional).*

Leader: As we sit quietly and focus on being here, let us clear our minds of where we have been and focus on being in this moment.

Opening Poem/Reading
Rather than a reading, show a 3-minute free downloadable relaxation video from www.meditainment.com called "Free Stress Buster Video." It can be downloaded once for unlimited viewing (registration required). The video is also available on YouTube (http://www. youtube.com/watch?v=YcK9MwwTDjI).

Introduce the video as a 3-minute exercise that will help participants relax their minds and become focused on preparing for the lesson. Let the group know that what we do in the next 3 minutes is an important sexual health in recovery tool. It is an excellent way to model skills for the lesson and to relax any group tension that may arise in anticipation of discussing nonconsensual sex. Do not process the experience. Move to introduction.

GROUP INTRODUCTION

Have a group member volunteer to read aloud.
Welcome to the sexual health in recovery group. We are here to talk about sex and how our sexual lives affect recovery from drug and alcohol addiction. Some people in recovery risk a relapse because of their sexual behavior at the treatment center or away from the treatment program. This is a place to talk about sexual behavior and sexual health so we can be abstinent from drugs and alcohol. It is also a place to learn about sexual behavior and situations that put men and women in recovery at risk for not completing this treatment program.

Sexual health in recovery is a time to talk about human sexuality and sexual health in a respectful and informed manner. We encourage everyone to be as honest and open as you can be. You are not required to reveal anything about your current or past sexual behavior that would be uncomfortable to discuss. It is important to listen to each other. For some of us, our sexual behavior is the most serious risk to staying in recovery. For others, our sexual behavior gets us into dangerous situations that are triggers to use or drink. A few of us may have little concern about how our sexual behavior contributes to relapse. This group is an opportunity for everyone to learn about the important connection between recovery and sexual health.

LESSON OBJECTIVE

Ask another group member to volunteer to read aloud.
The subject of today's sexual health in recovery group is nonconsensual sex and the high frequency of sexual abuse among men and women in treatment for drug and alcohol addiction. We will learn definitions for sexual abuse as well as correct common myths and assumptions about addiction and sexual abuse.

Women and men in recovery will increase their likelihood of staying sober when they can manage feelings linked with their history of nonconsensual sex. We will separate into two groups, one for men and the other for women. Each group will discuss common factors faced by sexual abuse survivors. We will focus on the importance of personal and physical safety as the necessary building blocks for becoming more aware of our own individual symptoms and feelings associated with sexual abuse or violence.

Each group will learn and practice together the "Self-Soothing Checklist." We will discuss the uses of the "Self-Soothing Checklist" to increase confidence in creating feelings of safety in our bodies and minds. Regulating our internal feeling state is vital preparation for looking more closely at a history of sexual pain and hurt. This is a very important skill that may increase your ability to sustain your early recovery and succeed with completing the treatment program.

LECTURE

Leader: As you can tell by our introductory portion of our class, today we are going to address an intense and emotion-filled topic. We are going to talk about how sex and sex acts can be used to hurt, terrify, control, or demean children, young people, and adults. I am imagining that some of you may already be having feelings just knowing we are going to talk about this subject. Let's take a few minutes and see what feelings people may be experiencing as we begin our topic of sexual abuse. We know when we are describing a feeling or an emotion when we can substitute the phrase "I am" rather than "I feel" and the sentence makes sense. For example "I feel that I don't want to be in this class" is restated as "I am don't want to be in this class." A feeling statement is "I feel tense and anxious about being in this class." Thus, "I am tense and anxious about being in this class" works as a sentence as well. The person has expressed a feeling. (The leader could prepare a list of feeling words for participants to use during the lesson. EQI.org has a continually growing list of feeling words.)

Call on participants who want to offer a feeling. Clarify if members use a thought or description of a situation. Encourage them to find a feeling word instead.

Leader: The most important guideline to remember about this session is that you only need to participate at the level where you feel safe. No one will be asked to reveal any personal information about his or her history or experience with sexual assault or sexual abuse. This class is not a support group for sexual abuse survivors. We will talk about the subject of sexual abuse and teach you valuable recovery skills. The tools are applicable for everyone in recovery regardless of whether she or he has a history of sexual trauma. The skills we are going to teach are particularly useful for sexual abuse survivors because they focus on regulating the sensations and feelings in your body.

Leader: Let's start by talking about why we are including a sexual abuse lesson in our classes on sex/drug-linked relapse prevention. What comes to mind as to why we may have included nonconsensual sex and sexual abuse in the sexual health in recovery program?

Invite people to share their thoughts and ideas. Reinforce perspectives that assume a higher frequency of sexual abuse, being a victim of nonconsensual sex, and/or forcing someone to have sex when using among chemically dependent people. Also reinforce that there is a higher risk for sexual trauma as a result of drug/alcohol addiction and for developing a drug/alcohol addiction in response to a childhood or adolescent sexual trauma. Thoughts and feelings about sexual abuse may be so overwhelming that they might trigger a craving to use to make the feelings go away.

Leader: As you can see by the answers in the group, many addicts in recovery need to address healing from past sexual trauma as part of their long-term recovery and prevention of relapse.

Sexual trauma can leave a scar that disrupts your sexuality. Before we break into separate groups, let's talk for a few minutes about what we mean by trauma and specifically what are the ways both men and women's sexual lives may be affected by sexual trauma.

In their book, *Sex Matters for Women*, Sallie Foley, Sally Kope, and Dennis Sugrue (2002) define trauma as a "shock that follows a disastrous or terrifying experience. Your brain and nervous system interpret the traumatic event as a life-or-death crisis. Your body goes into a self-protective mode, preparing you to defend yourself or to flee from the danger. Unfortunately, even after the real danger has passed, the traumatized mind and nervous system continue to respond, sometimes for years, as if the threat still exists" (Foley et al., 2002, p. 186). We can tell if our bodies and minds are still responding to the trauma in a variety of ways. Here are a few common self-protective measures in response to trauma:

1. Loss of interest in normal pursuits or interests (such as school, hobbies, friends, goals, sports, relationships) or loss of interest in things that were fun or enjoyable (such as music, movies, the arts).

2. Loss of interest in sex or pleasure (difficulty with sexual functioning, no interest in sex, unable to have orgasms).
3. Hypervigilance (being constantly on guard, looking for another threat, being highly reactive to unexpected sounds, sights, smells, touch, images).
4. Difficulty relaxing during sex, sleep, down times, alone times, night time.
5. Being in a heightened state of arousal (increased heart rate, sleep problems, anxiety, tension, panic, nervousness, and quick to startle). All of these feelings interfere with sexual desire and arousal.
6. A decrease in self-confidence.
7. Lack of trust in your own feelings or emotions.
8. The desire to suppress, deny, or repress feelings or to use drugs or alcohol to diminish or drown out intense or strong feelings. Of course some of the strong feelings you may be squashing may be sexual or erotic feelings.

Leader: Child sexual abuse is defined by the U.S. Department of Health and Human Services (2007) as: "The employment, use, persuasion, inducement, enticement, or coercion of any child to engage in, or assist any other person to engage in, any sexually explicit conduct or simulation of such conduct for the purpose of producing a visual depiction of such conduct; The rape, and in cases of caretaker or interfamilial relationships, statutory rape, molestation, prostitution, or other form of sexual exploitation of children, or incest with children."

Let's correct some possible sexual abuse misconceptions. One misconception is that child sexual abuse causes alcoholism or drug addiction. The truth is, many factors contribute to the connection between sexual abuse and addiction. Some of them are:

■ The severity, frequency, and intrusiveness of the abuse.
■ Family relationships prior to the abuse.
■ Family relationships after the abuse.
■ Preconceptions about reducing sexual anxieties by drinking or using.
■ Drinking and drug use of sexual partners.
■ Decline in economic status from childhood to adulthood.
■ Lack of adequate care, supervision, and protection as a child due to addictions in mother and father.

Leader: Child sexual abuse may be an important risk factor, but rarely (if ever) enough to cause an addiction. The National Institute on Drug Abuse identifies no single factor that determines the development of addiction to drugs (NIDA, 2008).

A more reasonable assumption is that child sexual abuse disrupts many aspects of childhood development. In adult life these disruptions in development may result in increased risk of low self-esteem, social and economic failure, social insecurity, difficulties with intimacy, and sexual problems. Using drugs and alcohol to cope with these adult difficulties may be a significant reason why so many addicts have a history of sexual abuse.

A second misconception is that women and men who experience sexual abuse will have similar reactions and consequences. Gender is key to how someone experiences sexual abuse or nonconsensual sex. Men and women will perceive, remember, and emotionally process sexual abuse and trauma differently. Women have some predictable ways of responding to trauma. Men also have separate and predictable ways of responding to trauma. We are now going to separate into two groups and spend the rest of our class discussing how women and men experience sexual trauma. Each group will learn some tools for increasing safety in our bodies when we feel intense feelings associated with past sexual abuse or sexual assault.

Divide men and women into two groups, and conduct the remainder of the lesson in separate rooms with separate facilitators. It is strongly recommended to have a man lead the men's group and a woman lead the women's group. Separate lessons for men's and women's group are provided.

MEN'S GROUP

Experiential Learning

Leader: Now that we are all settled into our group, let's start by reminding everyone of the boundaries we keep when we meet as separate groups. Who would like to remind us all about these boundaries?

Call on participants to reinforce the guidelines of privacy of these groups.

Leader: Thanks for the overview. Are there any questions or comments about our boundaries?

Address any issues raised by participants.

Leader: We are going to start by focusing on three types of nonconsensual sex. What I mean by nonconsensual is any sexual contact that involves force; being drugged or drunk, assaulted, bullied, intimidated, threatened, or terrorized; exploitation; or violation of boundaries without consent. We are going to discuss rape, child sexual abuse, and incest. We want to define each of these words.

Nonconsensual sex that involves the use of physical force or occurs when the person is unconscious is generally called rape. Rape is a situation either of brute force or threatening further harm to the person to force his or her consent to sex. Often a victim is given a choice to avoid death, terrible harm, or harm to loved ones such as children, spouse, or family if he or she cooperates with the forced sex. Questions that have been debated about defining rape continue to be clarified by the law, politicians, and sex experts. I do not want us to get too focused on debating these distinctions today. I do want to highlight that rape involves:

1. Sex
2. Force or threat of more harm unless victim consents
3. Minimum of two people: rape victim and rape perpetrator

Leader: Child sexual abuse refers to child and adult contact and interactions when the child is used for the sexual stimulation of the adult perpetrator or another person. A child, by definition or statute, is unable to give consent to this sexual interaction with the adult. There are three key areas to consider if you are unsure whether you experienced child sexual abuse. Child sexual abuse involves:

1. Contact between a child and an adult
2. Sexual contact between an adult and a child
3. Child used for sexual stimulation of adult

Leader: Incest can involve rape, sexual abuse, or it can be neither of these. Incest is best understood as sexual contact between relatives, family members, or persons who are culturally, legally, or customarily not considered as potential sex partners because of family or genetic relations.

We are going to look at these types of sexual trauma from the perspective of men. We know that the experience and the meaning of sexual trauma are different for boys and girls. Many things are similar, but some are different. What are the consequences for boys who experience sexual trauma when growing up? First of all, we know a lot more about what happens to girls than we do for boys. What do you think may be some of the reasons we know less about boys who have experienced sexual abuse?

Ask participants their ideas. Look for comments about the following:

- *Fears that disclosure of sexual abuse won't be believed*
- *Ideas that men are not supposed to be victims*
- *Fears that it won't be thought of as abuse if the perpetrator was a woman or a gay man introducing a gay adolescent into gay sex*
- *Fears that sexual abuse by a man may make a boy question his sexual orientation (the boy may be prematurely considered homosexual, the abuse may cause the boy to become homosexual)*
- *Fears that a man will be perceived as less masculine if he has experienced sexual abuse*

An additional purpose of these early discussions is to gradually get the group more comfortable with sitting with each other and discussing sexual trauma.

Leader: A high proportion of chemically dependent men have a history of sexual abuse. Not knowing what to do with this part of your history and how it fits into your overall sobriety and healing could be a significant risk for relapse or for not completing treatment. Sobriety will bring about remembering things you have wanted to forget. Being clean and sober gives you an opportunity to clear your mind and begin to get clarity about what lead you into drugs and alcohol as a coping solution. For many addicts, alcohol and drugs are a self-medication for the trauma associated with sexual abuse. Let's look for a bit at some of the common trauma consequences boys and men experience as a result of sexual trauma. First we will look at what children experience. Most of what we know about the initial effects of child sexual abuse in young children does not differ between girls and boys. Here is a brief outline of the effects.

Preschool
- Increased sexualized behavior
- Anxiety
- Nightmares

- Vigilance
- Bedwetting
- Depression
- Immaturity
- Overly dependent
- More impulsive

School Age

- Significantly less able to learn in school environment
- Immaturity
- Aggression
- Depression
- Perceived as more emotionally disturbed
- Wide range of fears
- Excessive masturbation
- Inappropriate places for masturbation
- Sexual aggression
- Sexualized behavior
- Increased frequency of school problems
- Early experimentation with alcohol, cigarettes, drugs

Adolescent

- Running away
- Alcohol abuse or dependency
- Drug abuse or dependency
- Sexually careless
- Sexually more adventurous
- High frequency of sexual mistakes
- Severe depression
- Low self-esteem
- Self-injury
- Suicidal thoughts
- Suicide attempts

Pause here to welcome comments about the information. Remind group that disclosing a personal history of abuse is not necessary or required when responding to the information. Remind participants that this lesson is about learning how to manage feelings in the body that may come up when focusing on the topic of sexual abuse. Encourage group members who express powerful feelings or emotions to take a deep breath and focus on relaxing.

Leader: Just because someone has experienced nonconsensual sex or abuse does not mean it results in the same emotional or behavioral consequences. However, adult men and women who survived childhood sexual abuse do report some significant differences in how they respond to and interpret the meaning of the abuse.

Now let's look at the differences between men and women survivors of sexual trauma. When we compare sexually abused women with non–sexually abused women, these are some of the differences.

Sexually Abused Women Compared With Non–Sexually Abused Women

Most Common Long-Term Effect Is Depression
- More severe levels of depression
- More frequent episodes of depression
- Increased risk for requiring hospitalization for depression if also sexually abused
- Increased risk of depression over one's lifetime
- Self-esteem problems intensify over time
- Higher risk of self-injury
- Higher risk of self-destructive behaviors

Another Common Long-Term Effect Is Anxiety
- More likely if force used
- More likely if abuse occurred with a family member

Relationship Difficulties
- Fear intimacy
- Higher frequency of sexual dysfunction
  - Especially if abuse is very severe
  - Especially if abuse was perpetrated by father or stepfather
- Increased risk for revictimization
  - Rape
  - Nonconsensual sex
  - Domestic violence

Leader: Conclusions about men are far less well-known, since most of the sexual abuse survivors studied are women. However, the things we do know are as follows.

Sexually Abused Men Compared
with Non–Sexually Abused Men
- Higher rate of depression
- Higher rate of anxiety
- Symptoms of trauma
- Poor self-esteem
- Higher frequency of self-medicating with alcohol and drugs
- Higher frequency of addiction to drugs and alcohol (women report higher frequency of depression and anxiety)
- Intense anger
- Sexual dysfunction
- Problems with intimacy

You may pause again to invite discussion of thoughts and feelings about the content without focusing on personal disclosure. Focus the group on learning the information and the feelings members are having about the information.

Leader: After taking into account the gender of the sexual abuse survivor, research has shown that the specific circumstances of the abuse are extremely significant in determining the long-term effects of the abuse. The more severe effects of child sexual abuse for men and women seemed to be correlated with several factors:

Was Force Used?
- Most significant of all factors
- The higher the force the higher the degree of trauma
- High levels of conflict in family
- Low level of family support
- May result in less self-blame for the abuse (this is a good thing)

What Is the Relationship With the Perpetrator?
- Trauma more severe if perpetrator was a father/mother or stepfather/stepmother
- Mental illness effects more severe if perpetrator was a father/mother or stepfather/stepmother
- How much trust was betrayed by the abuse?
  - In adults, the long-term trauma effect has more to do with how much the abuser was trusted by the victim.

- How much was the child seduced and persuaded by the perpetrator?
  - Was fear, extortion, threats of harm, blackmail, exchange for favors used?
- How much of a prior relationship did the child have with the perpetrator?

What Was the Duration of the Abuse?

- Some evidence of an increase in mental illness in adults the longer the abuse went on
- Increase in adult problems when abuse is a sexual contact rather than noncontact
  - Fondling of genitals, oral sex, sexual intercourse, use of objects more severe than kissing or clothed contact
- Children exhibited more traumatic outcomes in adulthood when their mothers demonstrated low support at the time abuse was disclosed.

Leader: OK, we just covered quite a bit of information. Some of you may have had some reactions or responses to the information. We are not going to have a personal disclosure discussion. What we are going to do is discuss how you can make it safer to be aware of the thoughts, feelings, memories, or awareness you may have about sexual trauma.

The most important area of safety if we were sexually abused is within our own bodies. Our bodies are where we felt and experienced the abuse. So it is within our bodies that we will focus on creating a safe place. When an addict in early recovery has a body sensation or feeling that does not feel safe, he may become afraid and want to stop the body feeling as soon as possible.

We want to teach you a few skills that are designed to provide a greater ability to regulate these body feelings. Being able to regulate body sensations and feelings is a foundation of safety within your body. Each of the skills will only take a minute or two. These skills can be practiced anywhere. They are portable. They do not cost anything. They do not require any special equipment. You have everything you need to use these tools right in your own body. All of these tools have one thing in common. They are self-soothing tools. What do you think we mean by "self-soothing"?

Ask group for definitions of self-soothing.

Leader: There are three aspects of self-soothing that our tools will focus on:

1. Safe environment
2. Comfort in body
3. Pleasing your senses

Leader: Let's all take a few minutes and talk about what makes an environment, the space that surrounds us, feel safe. What makes an environment feel safe for men?

Lead a brief discussion on a safe environment for men. Listen for examples that describe absence of threats, no risk of harm, predictable, lack of judgment, low risk of embarrassment or ridicule. Write the answers down on the board.

Leader: This is quite a list. As you can see, many things go into making an environment feel safe. I suggest that as you are trying to learn these self-soothing skills, you put yourself in a safe environment to practice them. Most people fail at self-soothing exercises because they do not practice them and wait until they need them. This puts too much pressure on the tool and will not let you get the benefit. So the first key is to practice these skills in a safe environment.

Topic Skill Practice

Leader: Not only is it important to move yourself to a safe environment to practice self-soothing, but you must also increase a feeling of safety inside your body as well. Comfort in your body is central to beginning to address the topic of sexual abuse. Taking a specific action to feel safe in your body is called self-soothing.

We are going to focus on a two-step approach to self-soothing. The first step is the check-in, followed by the second step, which is using one, two, three, or all four self-soothing tools. Both of these steps are necessary to benefit immediate self-soothing. I am handing out the "Self-Soothing Checklist." This is a tool that guides you through the self-soothing practice skills.

Hand out copies of "Self-Soothing Checklist" (Lesson 8 appendix, A).

Leader: The first step is to check for a safe environment. This list can be modified and changed by you as you learn what is important to you. This is a list of some basic elements of a safe environment. Add to the list circumstances that are important to you. The next step is to choose a self-soothing tool. Let's go over each of them one at a time and give you plenty of time to practice.

Go through each of the self-soothing tools (belly breathing, clasping your hands, tense-relax-breath-tense-relax-breath, and elephant hang) by having the group practice each step of each exercise and then put the exercise together. Have members who are familiar with any of the exercises give tips to others in the group. Encourage participants to share experiences with using any of these exercises. You should be very familiar with how to do each exercise before the lesson. Have fun with this part of the workshop. After sufficient practice with each these self-soothing exercises, move on to next step.

Leader: Another self-soothing exercises is not on the checklist. Instead of using our breath and body we are going to use our mind and imagination. We start by taking a moment to think about a mental image, a visual scene (either real or imagined) that you associate with comfort, letting go, and relaxation. This scene should not include drugs, alcohol, or sex. Let's all let our minds go for a minute and see what we come up with.

Pause for a minute to let people sit in quiet and ponder where their minds go.

Leader: OK, what did people think of or imagine in their minds?

Lead a discussion of the examples people share with the group.

Leader: Now that we have many ideas about the kinds of mental images that may be soothing, let's talk about why this is an important part of the self-soothing exercise. Remember that our topic is sexual trauma. Looking at our history of sexual hurts and pain will require us to prepare well in advance. We will need to stay sober and remain in recovery. We will need to develop basic trust and safety with our bodies and minds. Practicing this exercise in many different situations where we feel distress or overwhelming feelings can grow this trust. Knowing and believing that we have the ability to regulate, or turn down the heat, on an intense feeling or sensation will increase the personal and emotional safety for addressing sexual abuse.

I am passing around a 3 by 5 card for you to write two relaxation symbols on. On one side, write or draw your relaxation symbol or word. On the other side, do the same with a different symbol or word.

Hand out index cards to each member. Let this be a private moment for group members. Let them find this symbol or word on their own. This moment of autonomy and self-reflection is important for group members to experience. This is a time to discover an inner knowledge that is not dependent on the group. Encourage people to wait until something comes to mind. Do not rush the process. When participants have finished, return to leading group.

Leader: Now, fold this card up and place it in your pocket. I will give you several blank cards to make copies of this relaxation symbol card.

Hand out additional cards to each member.

Leader: You can take this with you wherever you go. Sometimes we will forget to think about these simple yet powerful tools to use our minds to assist our bodies to relax. You can use these relaxation symbols in conjunction with any of the self-soothing exercises or just all by itself. What might be some situations you could use your relaxation symbol all on its own?

Have a brief discussion of situations that the participants offer to share.

Leader: So you can see, having a mental tool to use can come in handy when a physical form of self-soothing is not available. Over time your body and mind will become less startled and tense when strong feelings emerge as an outcome of practicing these skills.

For those of you who want additional resources to read about healing from sexual abuse or learning more about sexual abuse, I have a handout listing a few books, organizations, and Web sites.

Hand out "Sexual Trauma Resource List."

Closing

Now let's take a moment to bring the workshop to a close. Let's take a moment to again quiet ourselves, take a deep breath to quiet our minds, our hearts, and our spirits. In this quiet place, remind yourself that we have to take a safe and comfortable pace to address a history of sexual trauma. Addicts in recovery have many things in common with each other. We have learned today that many of us share a history of sexual hurts and injuries in our childhood or even more recently before entering treatment. By practicing the self-soothing tool we can use not only our courage to face this part of our selves but also our bodies and minds to support us in this important work of recovery.

WOMEN'S GROUP

Experiential Learning

Leader: Now that we are all settled into our group, let's start by reminding everyone of the boundaries we keep when we meet as separate groups. Who would like to remind us all about these boundaries?

Call on participants to reinforce the guidelines of privacy of these groups.

Leader: Thanks for the overview. Are there any questions or comments about our boundaries?

Address any issues raised by participants.

Leader: We are going to start by focusing on three types of non-consensual sex. What I mean by non-consensual is any sexual contact that involves force, being drugged or drunk, assaulted, bullied, intimidated, threatened, and terrorized, exploitation or violation of boundaries without consent. We are going to discuss rape, child sexual abuse, and incest. We want to define each of these words.

Nonconsensual sex that involves the use of physical force or that occurs when the person is unconscious is generally called rape. Rape is a situation either of brute force or threatening further harm to the person to force his or her consent to sex. Often a victim is given a choice to avoid death, terrible harm, or harm to loved ones such as children, spouse, or family if he or she cooperates with the forced sex. Questions that have been debated about defining rape continue to be clarified by the law, politicians, and sex experts. I do not want us to get too focused on debating these distinctions today. I do want to highlight that rape involves:

1. Sex
2. Force or threat of more harm unless the victim consents
3. Minimum of two people: rape victim and rape perpetrator

Leader: Child sexual abuse refers to child and adult contact and interactions when the child is used for the sexual stimulation of the adult perpetrator or another person. A child, by definition or statute, is unable to give consent to this sexual interaction with the adult. There are three key areas to consider if you are unsure whether you experienced child sexual abuse. Child sexual abuse involves:

1. Contact between a child and an adult
2. Sexual contact between an adult and a child
3. Child used for sexual stimulation of adult

Leader: Incest can involve rape, sexual abuse, or it can be neither of these. Someone can experience any or all three of the terms we are defining. Incest is best understood as sexual contact between relatives, family members, or persons who are culturally, legally, or customarily not considered as potential sex partners because of family or genetic relations.

We are going to look at these types of sexual trauma from the perspective of women. We know that the experience of sexual trauma is different for boys than for girls. Many things are similar, but some things are different. What are the consequences for girls who experience sexual trauma when growing up?

Ask participants their ideas. Look for comments about the following:

■ *Fears of disclosure of sexual abuse not being believed*
■ *Being abused by a person in position of trust*
■ *Fears that it won't be thought of as abuse if the person was introducing you to gay sex*
■ *Thinking you may have allowed the abuse because it brought you attention that you craved*
■ *Feeling ashamed of how your body responded during the abuse, especially if you became aroused or had an orgasm*

An additional purpose of these early discussions is to gradually get the group more comfortable with sitting with each other and discussing sexual trauma.

Leader: Today we are going to talk about sexual abuse because such a high proportion of chemically dependent women have a history of sexual abuse. Not knowing what to do with this part of your history and how it fits into your overall sobriety and healing could be a significant risk for relapse or for not completing your treatment program. Sobriety will bring about memories of things you have wanted to forget. Being clean and sober gives you an opportunity to clear your mind and begin to get clarity about what lead you into drugs and alcohol as a coping solution. For many women, alcohol and drugs are a self-medication for the trauma associated with sexual abuse. Let's look for a bit at some of the common trauma consequences girls and women experience as a result of sexual trauma. First we will look at what children experience. Most of what we know about the initial effects of child sexual abuse in children does not differ between girls and boys. Here is a brief outline of the effects.

Preschool
- Increased sexualized behavior
- Anxiety
- Nightmares
- Vigilance
- Bedwetting
- Depression
- Immaturity
- Overly dependent
- More impulsive

School Age
- Significantly less able to learn in school environment
- Immaturity
- Aggression
- Depression
- Perceived as more emotionally disturbed
- Wide range of fears
- Excessive masturbation
- Inappropriate places for masturbation
- Sexual aggression
- Sexualized behavior
- Increased frequency of school problems
- Early experimentation with alcohol, cigarettes, drugs

Adolescent
- Running away
- Alcohol abuse or dependency
- Drug abuse or dependency
- Sexually careless
- Sexually more adventurous
- High frequency of sexual mistakes
- Severe depression
- Low self-esteem
- Self-injury
- Suicidal thoughts
- Suicide attempts

Leader takes pause here to welcome comments about the information. Remind group that disclosing personal history of abuse is not necessary or required when responding to the information. Remind participants that this lesson is about learning how to manage feelings in the body that may come up when focusing on the topic of sexual abuse. Leader will encourage group members who express feelings or emotions to take a deep breath and focus on relaxing.

Leader: Just because someone has experienced nonconsensual sex or abuse does not mean it results in the same emotional or behavioral consequences. However, adult women and men who survived childhood sexual abuse do report some significant differences in how they respond to and interpret the meaning of the abuse.

Now let's look at the differences between women and men survivors of sexual trauma. When we compare sexually abused women with non–sexually abused women, these are some of the differences.

Sexually Abused Women Compared With Non–Sexually Abused Women
Most Common Long-Term Effect Is Depression

- More severe levels of depression
- More frequent episodes of depression
- Increased risk for requiring hospitalization for depression if also sexually abused
- Increased risk of depression over one's lifetime
- Self-esteem problems intensify over time
- Higher risk of self-injury
- Higher risk of self-destructive behaviors

Another Common Long-Term Effect Is Anxiety
- More likely if force used
- More likely if abuse occurred with a family member

Relationship Difficulties
- Fear intimacy
- Higher frequency of sexual dysfunction
  - Especially if abuse is very severe
  - Especially if abuse was perpetrated by father or stepfather
- Increased risk for revictimization
  - Rape
  - Nonconsensual sex
  - Domestic violence

Leader: Conclusions about men are far less well-known, since most of the sexual abuse survivors studied are women. We do know some general information .

Sexually Abused Men Compared With Non–Sexually Abused Men
- Higher rate of depression
- Higher rate of anxiety
- Symptoms of trauma
- Poor self-esteem
- Higher frequency of self-medicating with alcohol and drugs
- Higher frequency of addiction to drugs and alcohol (women report higher frequency of depression and anxiety)
- Intense anger
- Sexual dysfunction
- Problems with intimacy

Pause again to invite discussion of thoughts and feelings about the content without focusing on personal disclosure. Keep the group focused on learning the information and the feelings members are having about the information.

Leader: After taking into account the gender of the sexual abuse survivor, research has shown that the specific circumstances of the abuse are extremely significant in determining the long-term effects of the abuse. The more severe effects of child sexual abuse for women and men seemed to be correlated with several factors.

Was Force Used?
- Most significant of all factors
- The higher the force, the higher degree of trauma
- High levels of conflict in family
- Low level of family support
- May result in less self-blame for the abuse (this is a good thing)

What Is the Relationship With the Perpetrator?
- Trauma more severe if perpetrator was a father/mother or stepfather/stepmother
- Mental illness effects more severe if perpetrator was a father/mother or stepfather/stepmother
- How much trust was betrayed by the abuse?
  - In adults, the long-term trauma effect has more to do with how much the abuser was trusted by the victim.
  - How much was the child seduced and persuaded by the perpetrator?
    - Was fear, extortion, threats of harm, blackmail, or exchange for favors used?
  - How much of a prior relationship did the child have with the perpetrator?

What Was the Duration of the Abuse?
- Some evidence of an increase in mental illness in adults the longer the abuse went on
- Increase in adult problems when abuse is a sexual contact rather than noncontact
  - Fondling of genitals, oral sex, sexual intercourse, use of objects more severe than kissing or clothed contact
- Children exhibited more traumatic outcomes in adulthood when their mothers demonstrated low support at the time abuse was disclosed

Leader: OK, we just covered quite a bit of information. Some of you may have had some reactions or responses to the information. We are not going to have a personal disclosure discussion. What we are going to do is discuss how you can make it safer to be aware of the thoughts, feelings, memories, or awareness you may have about sexual trauma.

The most important area of safety if we were sexually abused is within our own bodies. Our bodies are where we felt and experienced the abuse. So it is within our bodies that we will focus on creating a safe place. When a woman in early recovery has a body sensation or feeling that does not feel safe, she may become afraid and want to stop the body feeling as soon as possible. We want to teach you a few skills that are designed to provide a greater ability to regulate these body feelings. Being able to regulate body sensations and feelings is a foundation of safety within your body. Each of the skills will only take a minute or two. These skills can be practiced anywhere. They are portable. They do not cost anything. They are free. They do not require any special equipment. You have everything you need to use these tools right in your own body. All of these tools have one thing in common. They are self-soothing tools. What do you think we mean by "self-soothing"?

Ask group for definitions of self-soothing.

Leader: There are three aspects of self-soothing that our tools will focus on:

1. Safe environment
2. Comfort in body
3. Pleasing your senses

Leader: Let's all take a few minutes and talk about what makes an environment, the space that surrounds us, feel safe. What makes an environment feel safe for women?

Lead a brief discussion on a safe environment for women. Listen for examples that describe absence of threats, no risk of harm, predictable, lack of judgment, being listened to. Have participants describe safety. Write answers down on the board.

Leader: This is quite a list. As you can see, many things go into making an environment feel safe. I suggest that as you are trying to learn these self-soothing skills, you put yourself in a safe environment to practice them. Most people fail at self-soothing exercises because they do not practice them and wait until they need them. This puts too much pressure on the tool and will not let you get the benefit. So the first key is to practice these skills in a safe environment.

Topic Skill Practice

Leader: Not only is it important to move yourself to a safe environment to practice self-soothing, but we must also increase a feeling of safety inside our bodies as well. Comfort in our bodies is central to beginning to address the topic of sexual abuse. Taking a specific action to feel safe in our bodies is called self-soothing. We are going to focus on a two-step approach to self-soothing. The first step is the check-in, followed by the second step, which is using one, two, three, or all four self-soothing tools. Both of these steps are necessary to benefit immediate self-soothing. I am handing out the "Self-Soothing Checklist." This is a tool that guides you through the self-soothing practice skills.

Hand out copies of "Self-Soothing Checklist."

Leader: The first step is to check for a safe environment. This list can be modified and changed by you as you learn what is important to you. This is a list of some basic elements of a safe environment. Add to the list circumstances that are important to you. The next step is to choose a self-soothing tool. Let's go over each of them one at a time and give you plenty of time to practice.

Go through each of the self-soothing tools (belly breathing, clasp your hands, tense-relax-breath-tense-relax-breath, and elephant hang) by having the group practice each step of each exercise and then put the exercise together. Have members who are familiar with any of the exercises give tips to others in the group. Encourage participants to share experiences with using any of these exercises. You should be very familiar with how to do each exercise before the lesson. Have fun with this part of the workshop. After sufficient practice with each these self-soothing exercises, move on to next step.

Leader: Another self-soothing exercises is not on the checklist. Instead of using our breath and body we are going to use our mind and imagination. We start by taking a moment to think about a mental image, a visual scene (either real or imagined) that you associate with comfort, letting go, and relaxation. This scene should not include drugs, alcohol, or sex. Let's all let our minds go for a minute and see what we come up with.

Pause for a minute to let people sit in quiet and ponder where their minds go.

Leader: OK, what did people think of or imagine in their minds?

Lead a discussion of the examples people share with the group.

Leader: Now that we have many ideas about the kinds of mental images that may be soothing, let's talk about why this is an important part of the self-soothing exercise. Remember that our topic is sexual trauma. Looking at our history of sexual hurts and pain will require us to prepare well in advance. We will need to stay sober and remain in recovery. We will need to develop basic trust and safety with our bodies and minds. Practicing this exercise in many different situations where we feel distress or overwhelming feelings can grow this trust. Knowing and believing that we have the ability to regulate, or turn down the heat, on an intense feeling or sensation will increase the personal and emotional safety for addressing sexual abuse.

I am passing around a 3 by 5 card for you to write two relaxation symbols on. On one side, write or draw your relaxation symbol or word. On the other side, do the same with a different symbol or word.

Hand out index cards to each member. Let this be a private moment for group members. Let them find this symbol or word on their own. This moment of autonomy and self-reflection is important for group members to experience. This is a time to discover an inner knowledge that is not dependent on the group. Encourage people to wait until something comes to mind. Do not rush the process. When participants have finished return to leading group.

Leader: Now, fold this card up and place it in your pocket. I will give you several blank cards to make copies of this relaxation symbol card.

Hand out additional cards to each member.

Leader: You can take this with you wherever you go. Sometimes we will forget to think about these simple yet powerful tools to use our minds to assist our bodies to relax. You can use these relaxation symbols in conjunction with any of the self-soothing exercises or just all by itself. What might be some situations you could use your relaxation symbol all on its own?

Have a brief discussion of situations that the participants offer to share.

Leader: So you can see, having a mental tool to use can come in handy when a physical form of self-soothing is not available. Over time your body and mind will become less startled and tense when strong feelings emerge as an outcome of practicing these skills.

For those of you who want additional resources to read about healing from sexual abuse or learning more about sexual abuse, I have a handout listing a few books, organizations, and Web sites.

Hand out "Sexual Trauma Resource List."

Closing

Now let's take a moment to bring the workshop to a close. Let's take a moment to again quiet ourselves, take a deep breath to quiet our minds, our hearts, and our spirits. In this quiet place, remind yourself that we have to take a safe and comfortable pace to address a history of sexual trauma. Addicts in recovery have many things in common with each other. We have learned today that many of us share a history of sexual hurts and injuries in our childhood or even more recently before entering treatment. By practicing the self-soothing tool we can use not only our courage to face this part of our selves but also our bodies and minds to support us in this important work of recovery.

REFERENCES

Anderson, C., Teicher, H. L., Polcari, A., & Renshaw, P. (2002). Abnormal T2 relaxation time in the cerebellar vermis of adults sexually abused in childhood: Potential role of the vermis in stress-enhanced risk for drug abuse. *Psychoneuroendocrinology* 27(1–2), 231–244.

Bass, E., & Davis, L. (1993). *Beginning to heal.* New York: HarperCollins.

Center for Substance Abuse Treatment. (2006). *Helping yourself heal: A Recovering Woman's Guide to Coping With the Effects of Childhood Abuse. DHHS Publication No. (SMA) 03–3789. Rockville, MD: Substance Abuse and Mental Health Services Administration.*

Foley, S., Kope, S., & Sugrue, D. (2002). *Sex matters for women: A complete guide to taking care of your sexual self.* New York: The Guildford Press.

Hein, S. (2009). Emotional Intelligence. Retrieved from http://eqi.org

Kendler, K. S., Bulik, C. M., Silberg, J., Hettema, J. M., Myers, J., Prescott, C. A., et al. (2000). Childhood sexual abuse and adult psychiatric and substance use disorders in women: An epidemiological and co-twin control analysis. *Archives of General Psychiatry, 57*(10), 953–959.

Lew, M. (1989). Victims no longer. Walnut Creek, CA: Launch Press.

National Institute of Drug Abuse (NIDA). (2008). *Drugs, brains and behavior: The science of addiction. Drug abuse and addiction.* Retrieved March 6, 2009, from http://www.drugabuse.gov/scienceofaddiction/addiction.html

Rosellini, G. (2002). *A women's guide to sex and recovery.* Retrieved March 6, 2009,from http://www.doitnow.org/pdfs/807.pdf

Swan, N. (1998). Exploring the role of child abuse in later drug abuse. *NIDA Notes, 13*(2). Retrieved May 22, 2009, from http://www.drugabuse.gov/NIDA_Notes/NNVol13N2.exploring.html

U.S. Department of Health and Human Services. (2007). *Definitions of child abuse and neglect.* Retrieved March 6, 2009,from http://www.childwelfare.gov/systemwide/laws_policies/statutes/define.cfm

Wendy Maltz: Healing our sexuality. (2009). PersonalLifeMedia.com (Episode 27). Retrieved May 23, 2009, from http://personallifemedia.com/podcasts/222-sex-love-and-intimacy

Wertheimer, A. (2003). *Consent to sexual relations.* Cambridge: Cambridge University Press.

LESSON 8 APPENDIX

A. Self-Soothing Checklist

Purpose

This tool can be used anytime you need to take a minute or two to relax and gather your thoughts. It can be useful if you are having feelings that upset, concern, or frighten you. Knowing you have the ability to change how you feel in your body may help you be more effective in approaching whatever early recovery situation you may find yourself in.

Directions

Check in with your thoughts and feelings. Do not judge or criticize yourself for these sensations. Put a check mark next to each current thought or body sensation.

_____ Heart beating faster

_____ Rapid thoughts in mind

_____ Imagining a catastrophe or frightening thing will happen

_____ Feeling ashamed or embarrassed

_____ Feeling hopeless

_____ Feeling discouraged

_____ Feeling afraid

_____ Thoughts flooded, cannot think clearly

_____ Thoughts of using

_____ Thoughts of fleeing to just get away

_____ Thoughts of hitting or hurting someone

_____ Memory of sexual abuse or trauma that I can't stop thinking about

_____ Memory of being hurt or injured that I can't stop thinking about

_____ Memory of being high that I can't stop thinking about

Rate the intensity level of your body sensations (1 = lowest to 10 = highest)

Circle one number 1   2   3   4   5   6   7   8   9   10

Do one or several self-soothing exercises.

Belly Breathing
- Place the palm of one hand on your belly and the palm of the other hand on your chest.
- Breathe through your nose and out your mouth.
- Take deep slow breaths by using your diaphragm.
- Deep breaths will move your lower palm out, with little movement from the palm on chest.
- Do this for several minutes.
- Imagine the breath coming in relaxing you and the breath going out releasing your distress.

Clasp Your Hands
- Stand straight.
- Cross left ankle over your right ankle.
- Stretch arms over your head.
- Cross right wrist over left wrist.
- Turn hands so palms are touching.
- Clasp your fingers.
- Twist hands down and toward your ribs.
- Rest hands on chest.
- Hold position for 2 minutes while breathing through your nose.

Tense-Relax-Breath-Tense-Relax-Breath
- Sit in a chair with your feet on the floor or lay on your back on the floor.
- Briefly tense each of the body parts in order: feet, lower legs, thighs, buttock, pelvis, abdomen, lower back.
- After each brief moment of hard tension, release the tension completely and feel the muscle soften and relax.

- Briefly tense each body part in order: hands, forearms, upper arms and shoulders, belly, back, neck, face.
- Now take some deep breaths and imagine tension leaving your body when you breathe out.
- Repeat.

Elephant Hang

- Stand straight, shoulders back, arms at your sides.
- Keep your knees straight; slowly and gently bend at the waist with your arms moving toward your toes.
- Stop at a 90-degree angle.
- Gently sway your arms back and forth.
- Take deep breaths.
- Slowly raise back to starting position.
- Repeat.

Re-rate the intensity level of your body sensations (1 = lowest to 10 = highest)

Circle one number 1   2   3   4   5   6   7   8   9   10

B. Sexual Trauma Resource List

National Suicide Prevention Lifeline, 800-273-8255 or 800-799-4889 (TTY)

National Clearinghouse on Child Abuse and Neglect Information, nccanch.acf.hhs.gov, 800-394-3366

National Clearinghouse for Alcohol and Drug Information (NCADI), www.ncadi.samhsa.gov, 800-729-6686, or 800-487-4889 (TDD)

Substance Abuse Treatment Facility Locator, www.findtreatment.samhsa.gov, 800-662-HELP

National Mental Health Information Center, www.mentalhealth.samhsa.gov, 800-789-2647

Adult Children of Alcoholics, www.adultchildren.org, 310-534-1815

Co-Dependents Anonymous (CoDA), www.codependents.org, 602-277-7991

Emotions Anonymous International, www.emotionsanonymous.org, 651-647-9712

National Clearinghouse on Child Abuse and Neglect Information, www.calib.com/nccanch, 800-394-3366

National Mental Health Association, www.nmha.org, 800-969-6642

National Mental Health Consumers' Self-Help Clearinghouse, www.mhselfhelp.org, 800-553-4539

Parents Anonymous, www.parentsanonymous-natl.org, 909-621-6184

Posttraumatic Stress Disorder Alliance, www.ptsdalliance.org, 877-507-PTSD

Sidran Institute, www.sidran.org/resourcesurv.html, 410-825-8888

Survivors of Incest Anonymous, Inc., www.siawso.org, 410-893-3322

List compiled from: Center for Substance Abuse Treatment. Helping Yourself Heal: A Recovering Woman's Guide to Coping With the Effects of Childhood Abuse. DHHS Publication No. (SMA) 03–3789. Rockville, MD: Substance Abuse and Mental Health Services Administration, 2003.

Center for Substance Abuse Treatment (2006).

9   Out-of-Control Sexual Behavior

CORE CONCEPT

Men and women in early recovery may be disappointed to discover that abstinence from drugs and alcohol is not the end of their troubling or problematic sexual behavior. Although more strongly associated with men, concerns about sexual behavior are more commonly found among recovering addicts than in the general population (Braun-Harvey, 1997). Highly motivated men and women relapse because of untreated out-of-control sexual behavior (OCSB). This class will not determine if participants' sexual behavior is out of control. The primary purpose is to provide accurate information about compulsive sexual behavior as well as the role of untreated compulsive sexual behavior in relapse. We will deal with the consequences of premature conclusions about compulsive sexual behavior. This curriculum will present four core symptoms for problematic sexual behavior to the entire class. Specific symptoms among men and women will be the focus of separate groups. Each group will learn how to use the "Sexual Symptoms in Recovery Worksheet" to measure the severity of problematic sexual behavior and link these concerns with risk for relapse.

BELIEF STATEMENT

Sexual health in recovery is the ability to have accurate information about the signs and symptoms for out of control sexual behavior.

OBJECTIVES

Participants will
- Discuss behaviors and thinking patterns associated with OCSB.
- Link risks for relapse in sobriety and untreated OCSB.
- Practice using the "Sexual Symptoms in Recovery Worksheet."

CHANGE GOALS

- Distinguish relapse risk associated with OCSB.
- Assess and measure risk associated with unaddressed OCSB patterns.
- Understand link between relapse risk in recovery and unaddressed OCSB.
- If necessary, seek professional treatment or attend self-help programs for OCSB.

REQUIRED READING FOR GROUP LEADER

For this lesson the leader needs to be up-to-date on current theories and approaches for evaluating OCSB. Most important is for the leader not to use the language of one exclusive theory or approach to dealing with OCSB symptoms. Three sources provide an overview of the last 20 years in the development of theory and treatment for OCSB.

- In 1997, I wrote "Sexual Dependence Among Recovering Substance-Abusing Men" (Braun-Harvey, 1997). This chapter reviews theoretical conceptualizations of compulsive sexual behavior, sexual addiction, and hyperphilia as well as the interactive influences between substance abuse and OCSB.

■ Jack Morin's *The Erotic Mind* (1995) explores three types of erotic problems. In his chapter "When Turn-Ons Turn Against You" (pp. 171–202), he identifies "how the same emotions that intensify arousal can also produce unwanted side effects that inhibit our desire or disrupt our capacity for arousal and orgasm" (pp. 172–173). An important factor in sex/drug-linked behavior for some women and men in recovery is missing the opportunity to control negative feelings to increase or decrease arousal. He also identifies how "troublesome attractions" (p. 173) lead women and men to partners who will hurt or consistently let us down. Women in particular will identify with loving and desiring a partner with such intensity that they tolerate enormous pain to sustain the benefits of the attraction. Last, Morin looks at a very common dilemma for men in recovery with symptoms of OCSB: men who find it almost impossible or at best extremely difficult to experience love and passion with the same person. Men with OCSB symptoms may use drugs to resolve this conflict by taking, for example, crystal meth to feel intense arousal with someone they have no emotional connection with. When they are with someone they feel in love with, they have difficulty sustaining any sexual interest past a few initial sexual experiences. Understanding these dynamics will be valuable in listening to both men and women discuss their reactions to the lesson.

■ Last, leaders need to read "Sexual Addiction, Sexual Compulsivity, Sexual Impulsivity, or What? Toward a Theoretical Model" (Bancroft & Vukadinovic, 2004). Bancroft and Vukadinovic, sex researchers at The Kinsey Institute, suggest that OCSB "results from a variety of mechanisms" (p. 235) and conclude that attempting to consider an overriding definition for patterns of OCSB is premature until a much better understanding of what determines these behavior patterns has been established. They concur with the concept of compulsivity and addiction having treatment and clinical value for people living with the symptoms, but do not agree that these concepts generally explain the wider general class of the behaviors.

These three sources will provide a foundation for a more sex-positive, less quick-to-label discussion about OCSB. Reading these sources provides the leader with a language of behavior, actions, consequences, and feelings without resorting to overarching labels and diagnosis that, when prematurely attached to a discussion of sexual behavior, result in a barrier to curiosity and may establish an either/or attitude about OCSB symptoms (e.g., "Am I a sex addict or not?").

RECOMMENDED MATERIALS FOR GROUP LEADER

Becoming familiar with the variety of sexual recovery 12-step programs is essential. Knowing the distinctions between The Augustine Fellowship of Sex and Love Addicts Anonymous (SLAA) (http://www.slaafws.org), Sexual Compulsive Anonymous (http://www.sca-recovery.org), Sex Addicts Anonymous (http://www.sexaa.org), and Sexaholics Anonymous (www.sa.org) is necessary before leading this lesson.

Each program understands OCSB slightly (or in some cases, significantly) differently. For example, Sexaholics Anonymous (SA) sees lust as the sexual equivalent of alcohol for an alcoholic. Thus, abstinence from lust is a similar sobriety as abstinence from alcohol is for an alcoholic. SA defines sexual sobriety as "no sex with ourselves and no sex with any partner other than the spouse" (Sexaholics Anonymous [SA], 1989, p. 4). Any sex outside of heterosexual marriage, including masturbation is not abstinent from lust and outside the definition of Sexaholics Anonymous recovery. On the other hand, Sex and Love Addicts Anonymous views the range of OCSB as "a compulsive need for sex, extreme dependency on one or many people, or a chronic preoccupation with romance, intrigue, or fantasy" (Sex and Love Addicts Anonymous [SLAA], 1986). Sobriety in SLAA is "willingness to stop acting out in our own personal bottom-line addictive behavior on a daily basis" (SLAA, 1986). Masturbation, unmarried sexual partners, and same-sex partners are included in sexual sobriety.

REQUIRED MATERIALS FOR THE LESSON

- An mp3 player and music selection
- Blackboard, white board, or flip chart
- "Sexual Symptoms in Recovery Worksheet" (one copy for each participant) (Lesson 9 appendix)
- Computer with projector
- Sexual recovery 12-step fellowship orientation materials, local meeting schedules, and Web address information (to be compiled by group leader in advance)

OPENING

Opening Music: *Have quiet music playing as participants enter the room and ready themselves (optional).*

Leader: As we sit quietly and focus on being here, let us clear our minds of where we have been and focus on being in this moment.

Opening Poem/Reading:

Among men, sex sometimes results in intimacy; among women, intimacy sometimes results in sex.

—Barbara Cartland

Nobody dies from lack of sex. It's lack of love we die from.

—Margaret Atwood, *The Handmaid's Tale*

GROUP INTRODUCTION

Have a group member volunteer to read aloud.

Welcome to the sexual health in recovery group. We are here to talk about sex and how our sexual lives affect recovery from drug and alcohol addiction. Some people in recovery risk a relapse because of their sexual behavior at the treatment center or away from the treatment program. This is a place to talk about sexual behavior and sexual health so we can be abstinent from drugs and alcohol. It is also a place to learn about sexual behavior and situations that put men and women in recovery at risk for not completing this treatment program.

Sexual health in recovery is a time to talk about human sexuality and sexual health in a respectful and informed manner. We encourage everyone to be as honest and open as you can be. You are not required to reveal anything about your current or past sexual behavior that would be uncomfortable to discuss. It is important to listen to each other. For some of us, our sexual behavior is the most serious risk to staying in recovery. For others, our sexual behavior gets us into dangerous situations that are triggers to use or drink. A few of us may have little concern about how our sexual behavior contributes to relapse. This group is an opportunity for everyone to learn about the important connection between recovery and sexual health.

LESSON OBJECTIVE

Ask another group member to volunteer to read aloud.

The purpose of today's sexual health in recovery group is to learn about signs and symptoms for out-of-control sexual behavior. Today's class will empower you with introductory information about the link between out-of-control sexual behavior and relapse. We will identify common behaviors, thoughts, and perceptions for men and women with significant symptoms of problematic sexual behavior. Women and men in recovery increase their likelihood of staying sober when they have accurate information about the signs and symptoms for out-of-control sexual behavior.

We will not determine if your sexual behavior is out of control. We will discuss how people may rush to judgment and prematurely label sexual mistakes and poor sexual decision in early recovery as sex addiction. The entire class will learn four general symptoms for out-of-control sexual behavior.

Women and men experience symptoms of problematic sexual behavior, so we will spend the last section of the class in our separate men and women groups to discuss these symptoms in more detail. We will learn how to measure symptoms for out-of-control sexual behavior as a relapse prevention tool. We will briefly review a variety of resources, both online and within the 12-step community, to explore and address concerns about out-of-control sexual behavior.

LECTURE

Leader: Today's topic, sexual behavior that may be out of control, can be a source of many emotions, opinions, and uncomfortable memories. We begin by establishing some boundaries to make this topic a safe and respectful class discussion. There are four specific boundaries to highlight.

1. Our class is not focused on disclosing details about sexual behavior before recovery.
2. You are not required to discuss any aspect of your sexual history that you do not want to disclose.
3. We are not going to diagnose or assess if anyone has out-of-control sexual behavior, sexual addiction, love addiction, or compulsive sexual behavior.

4. We will use the term "OCSB" (which is shorthand for out-of-control sexual behavior) This is a term that is not a diagnosis or label. It is a way to describe a cluster of behaviors. You can use whatever term you are comfortable with. Using terms in this class is not labeling yourself or diagnosing yourself.

Leader: We are going to spend some time together in our large group going over exactly what OCSB looks like. We will pay particular attention to the relapse risks for people in recovery when they have insufficient information about OCSB or have not been assessed for OCSB. We will spend the remainder of the time in our separate men's and women's groups. Men and women experience OCSB differently. We want to give the men and the women time to go over symptoms of problematic sexual behavior.

How many of you have ever been to a class about OCSB? It might have been called compulsive or addictive sexual behavior.

Have a show of hands, allow people to share when, where, and so forth that they had some previous contact with this topic.

Leader: How many of you know someone who is in recovery for compulsive sexual behavior or sex addiction?

Have a show of hands; some people may want to comment or share something about who the person is and so forth.

Leader: What kind of sexual behaviors or sexual concerns do men and women who say they are sex addicts talk about?

Lead a brief discussion of behaviors. Focus on specific behaviors such as the following:

- *Spending too much time pursuing sex*
- *Having embarrassing negative consequences*
- *Losing a relationship because of online sex*
- *Paying for sex*
- *Having affairs*
- *Having sex with people you don't know or care about*
- *Having sex with people who will supply you with drugs*
- *Having sex with people who were high*
- *Making promises to stop a certain sexual behavior and not succeeding*

- *Thinking about sex all the time*
- *Seeing people as only sex objects*
- *Obsessing over a particular person*

Leader: We are going to focus on four common symptoms for all men and women living with OCSB. We will review what each of the four symptoms means and then we will divide into men and women's groups to discuss the four symptoms in more detail. Before ending we will practice using the "Sexual Symptoms in Recovery Worksheet."

The four symptoms are:

1. Sexual urges
2. Sexual thoughts
3. Conflicted ambivalence about sexual behavior
4. Direct emotional and personal consequences from sexual behavior

Leader: The first symptom is sexual urges. A sexual urge is intense sexual emotional or physical energy that drives someone to act or behave sexually. People with OCSB report extremely intense sexual urges. There urges happen often or even constantly throughout the day, and people can spend many hours a day or over a week's time preoccupied with these intense and frequent sexual urges. An urge is a physical and mental surge in both mind and body. A sexual urge is a sense of needing to do something quickly, urgently, and without much time to think about the behavior. An urge is such a strong feeling that the person is focused more on turning down the urge. People with OCSB tend to impulsively or desperately engage in sexual behavior to quiet the urge.

The second symptom is sexual thoughts: imagining, planning, and anticipating problematic sexual behavior. Women and men with OCSB focus a lot of their mental attention on sexual desires, memories, and activities. Thoughts about their worrisome sexual behavior are difficult to control. They are thinking about sexual behavior so much they experience a loss of control over their own thinking. It is common for men and women to report many hours a day and over 20 hours a week just thinking about or making plans for engaging in their problematic sexual urges.

The third symptom is ambivalence. Women and men with OCSB eventually become conflicted about their behavior. The most common complaint is spending too much time pursuing sex or relationships: time spent feeling sexual tension and excitement, anticipating, imagining, fantasizing, preparing, making time, and then actually doing the sexual behavior. All of this behavior takes time and can result in a distressing mixture of worry, uncertainty, conflict, emotional strain, anticipation, and hopeful relief or resignation in the moment of certainty just before engaging in the activity. Paradoxically, the anticipated excitement and pleasure that is imagined is far greater than the pleasure of the actual sex. This disappointment is an almost universal complaint of women and men with OCSB symptoms. Reality cannot live up to the fantasy. This disappointment leads to jumping back into the same behavior or making a promise not to do that again.

The fourth symptom is the consequences that result from OCSB—both emotional and personal. Emotional distress, shame, guilt, embarrassment, fear, anxiety, mental suffering, psychological pain, and emotional torment can result from OCSB. For men and women in early recovery, these emotional consequences from OCSB may be the single most serious risk for relapse. The emotions may trigger thoughts of using or drinking. Personal trouble—problems, chaos, damage, personal drama in relationships, marriage, family, and/or the workplace—can all be connected with OCSB symptoms. In early recovery, these painful consequences can trigger defeated attitudes that may increase risk of drinking or using. Financial, legal medical, physical, and mental health problems are additional consequences that stem directly for OCSB.

EXPERIENTIAL LEARNING

Leader: Before we separate into men's and women's groups, let's spend just a few minutes talking about a common problem in early recovery regarding OCSB symptoms. This is the problem of immediately labeling sexual mistakes in recovery as sexual addiction or compulsive sexual behavior. Early recovery can be a time where women and men make poor sexual decisions. Perhaps they ended up having sex with someone they really did not want to have sex with. They tell their sponsor about it and their sponsor focuses right away on whether or not they may need to go to a sexual addiction recovery group. Perhaps you just can't leave a relationship that you know is harmful. When you start talking about this, your friend encourages to consider a sex and love addicts meeting. What are some examples of sexual mistakes that could be prematurely labeled as sexual addiction?

Have a discussion about the examples people give. Keep the focus on why the example is a premature conclusion. Perhaps ask what could be other explanations for the sexual behavior? See if people are able to think a little less either/or, less black and white, about sexual mistakes.

Leader: The sexual health in recovery program hopefully provides tools to prevent clients from having to leave this treatment program as a consequence of a sexual mistake. We are trying to provide you with information as well as a place to discuss concerns about OCSB in the hope that people who need to discuss this more will be given information and opportunities to get the help they may need so they can stay sober.

The pattern we want to emphasize is someone using one situation, one mistake, one poor decision and concluding that the person must be a sex addict. It would be like concluding that anyone who ever drinks and drives, even if he or she is never caught, is an alcoholic. No one situation, no one behavior pattern means someone is compulsively sexual. The important thing to remember is that for there to be a serious concern about OCSB, there needs to be a pattern of out-of-control behavior, a long series of sexual situations and behaviors that result in shame, humiliation, secrecy, or harm. The person must also have a pervasive mental preoccupation about sex and sexual fantasy. All of these must fit together in a pattern.

We will spend the rest of the class in separate groups where we will discuss these four symptoms in the lives of men and women in recovery.

Divide into men's and women's groups. Each group should move to a private room with at least one group leader. The two small groups will not return to the larger group. The remainder of the session is conducted within the two groups.

WOMEN'S GROUP

Topic Skill Practice

Leader: We are going to spend some of the class giving you all a chance to discuss symptoms of OCSB for women. We are going to use the "Sexual Symptoms in Recovery Worksheet" to guide the discussion.

Hand out the "Sexual Symptoms in Recovery Worksheet" (Lesson 9 appendix).

Leader: Notice there are 12 items on the form. The four symptom areas we discussed in the large group are the focus of this worksheet. Items 1–4 deal with urges. Items 5–7 deal with thinking, 8–10 address problematic sexual behavior, and the last two items deal with consequences, both emotional and personal, that are a direct result of the problematic sexual behavior.

At the top of the form are the directions and space to write in the specific problematic sexual behavior that is being measured. What are some examples of problematic sexual behavior you might write in here? Remember, this class does not require or expect personal disclosure. You can give examples without it having to be about yourself.

Lead a 5-minute discussion. Ask participants to be specific, use details, set limits on vague or metaphorical statements. Vague statements are "I act out all the time," "I get my sex fix," "I get high from sex," "I fall in love way too easy," and "I can't get enough of it." Notice when statements are made in this vague way we have no idea what the actual behavior is or what negative consequences are linked with the behavior. Ask participants to clarify their examples with specific sexual and behavioral descriptions. This is an important sexual health group skill. Specific behavior and consequences, when spoken, will bring emotion and clarity. Being specific is an opportunity for shame processing and shame reduction. Language and words when spoken with others in a supportive environment help participants face the shame and move through the feelings associated with the details.

Have a member of the group read the first item aloud. Have the group discuss what the question is about. This is another moment for shame reduction processing. Have group members restate the meaning of the item to be rated. Members will use a variety of terms and descriptions that will be important for each person to say aloud and for others to listen to. This group exchange, grounded in reaction to the statements on the "Sexual Symptoms in Recovery Worksheet," provides a good container for risk taking within parameters that will keep the group focused.

This is a good time to discuss key terms like urges, strength of urges, and the distinction between a mild, moderate, and extreme urge. Go through all four urge items with the same process. A key point for facilitation is for members to use specific language and examples and to provide time to clarify what each item is asking and what women may experience who rate themselves in the 3–4 range. With each item the key question is: How might a high score on items related to sexual urges related to problematic sexual behavior be a relapse risk for a woman in early recovery? Repeat this same process with the remaining three topic areas.

Leader: The "Sexual Symptoms in Recovery Worksheet" can be filled out weekly or whenever you or a person in your personal support system recommends taking a look at a specific problematic sexual behavior. Looking at problematic sexual behavior symptoms before they trigger a high risk for relapse is an important sexual health in recovery skill.

What questions, comments, thoughts, observations, opinions, or feelings do you have about this worksheet and the symptoms of OCSB?

Facilitate a discussion that continues patterns of specific behavior and related consequences. Have group members be specific in language when discussing sexual behavior patterns. Integrate discussion of the four different 12-step fellowship programs into the discussion. Have information from each of the fellowships available for people to read. Have Web addresses available. If possible, have Web sites on a computer to show the various descriptions and meeting schedules in your local area.

Use the 12 items from the "Sexual Symptoms in Recovery Worksheet" to ground the conversation. The skill practice is to provide an opportunity to discuss compulsive or addictive sexual issues. Remember, this is not a diagnostic exercise. It is an opportunity to see if concerns about OCSB may need to be addressed as part of the participants' overall recovery.

Closing

Leader: Now let's take a moment to bring the workshop to a close. Let's take a moment to again quiet ourselves, take a deep breath to quiet our minds, our hearts, and our spirits. In this quiet place, remind yourself how valuable it is to take the time to be honest, vulnerable, and committed to recovery. As you leave the group today, remind yourself that a satisfying sexual life is a vital and important part of recovery. The self-reflection and tools you learned today may become an important part of maintaining your recovery.

MEN'S GROUP

Topic Skill Practice

Leader: We are going to spend some of the class giving you all a chance to discuss symptoms of OCSB for men. We are going to use the "Sexual Symptoms in Recovery Worksheet" to guide the discussion.

Hand out the "Sexual Symptoms in Recovery Worksheet."

Leader: Notice there are 12 items on the form. The four symptom areas we discussed in the large group are the focus of this worksheet. Items 1–4 deal with urges. Items 5–7 deal with thinking, 8–10 address problematic sexual behavior, and the last two items deal with consequences, both emotional and personal, that are a direct result of the problematic sexual behavior.

At the top of the form are the directions and space to write in the specific problematic sexual behavior that is being measured. What are some examples of problematic sexual behavior you might write in here? Remember, this class does not require or expect personal disclosure. You can give examples without it having to be about yourself.

Lead a 5-minute discussion. Ask participants to be specific, use details, set limits on vague or metaphorical statements. Vague statements are "I act out all the time," "I get my sex fix," "I get high from sex," "I hook up with people online," "I watch porn," "I can't get enough of it." Notice when statements are made in this vague way we have no idea what the actual behavior is or what negative consequences are linked with the behavior. Ask participants to clarify their examples with specific sexual and behavioral descriptions. This is an important sexual health group skill. Specific behavior and consequences, when spoken, will bring emotion and clarity. Being specific is an opportunity for shame processing and shame reduction. Language and words when spoken with others in a supportive environment help participants face the shame and move through the feelings associated with the details.

Have a member of the group read the first item aloud. Have group discuss what the question is about. This is another moment for shame reduction processing. Have group members restate the meaning of the item to be rated. Members will use a variety of terms and descriptions that will be important for each person to say aloud and for others to listen to. This group exchange, grounded in reaction to the statements on the "Sexual Symptoms in Recovery Worksheet" provides a good container for risk taking within parameters that will keep the group focused.

This is a good time to discuss key terms like urges, strength of urges, and the distinction between a mild, moderate, and extreme urge. Go through all four urges with the same process. A Key point for facilitation is for members to use specific language and examples and to provide time to clarify what each item is asking and what men may experience who rate themselves in the 3–4 range. With each item the key question is: How might a high score on items related to sexual urges related to problematic sexual behavior be a relapse risk for men in early recovery? Repeat this same process with the remaining three topic areas.

Leader: The "Sexual Symptoms in Recovery Worksheet" can be filled out weekly or whenever you or a person in your personal support system recommends taking a look at a specific problematic sexual behavior. Looking at problematic sexual behavior symptoms before they trigger a high risk for relapse is an important sexual health in recovery skill.

What questions, comments, thoughts, observations, opinions, or feelings do you have about this worksheet and the symptoms of OCSB?

Facilitate a discussion that continues patterns of specific behavior and related consequences. Have group members be specific in language when discussing sexual behavior patterns. Integrate discussion of the four different 12-step fellowship programs into the discussion. Have information from each of the fellowships available for people to read. Have Web addresses available. If possible, have Web sites on a computer to show the various descriptions and meeting schedules in your local area.

Use the 12 items from the "Sexual Symptoms in Recovery Worksheet" to ground the conversation. The skill practice is to provide an opportunity to discuss compulsive or addictive sexual issues. Remember, this is not a diagnostic exercise. It is an opportunity to see if concerns about OCSB may need to be addressed as part of the participants' overall recovery.

Closing

Leader: Now let's take a moment to bring the workshop to a close. Let's take a moment to again quiet ourselves, take a deep breath to quiet our minds, our hearts, and our spirits. In this quiet place, remind yourself how valuable it is to take the time to be honest, vulnerable, and committed to recovery. As you leave the group today, remind yourself that a satisfying sexual life is a vital and important part of recovery. The self-reflection and tools you learned today may become an important part of maintaining your recovery.

REFERENCES

Atwood, M. (2006). *The handmaid's tale*. New York: Random House.

Bancroft, J., & Vukadinovic, Z. (2004). Sexual addiction, sexual compulsivity, sexual impulsivity, or what? Toward a theoretical model. *Journal of Sex Research, 41*(3), 225–234.

Braun-Harvey, D. (1997). Sexual dependence among recovering substance-abusing men. In S. Straussner & L. Zelvin (Eds.), *Gender and addictions: Men and women in treatment* (pp. 359–384). Northvale, NJ: Jason Aronson.

Cartland, B. (n.d.). *Barbara Cartland quotes.* Retrieved March 7, 2009, from http://einstein/quotes/barbara_cartland/

Morin, J. (1995). *The erotic mind.* New York: HarperCollins.

Raymond, N., Lloyd, M., Miner, M., & Kim, S. W. (2007). Preliminary report on the development and validation of the sexual symptom assessment scale. *Sexual Addiction & Compulsivity, 14*(2), 119–129.

Sexaholics Anonymous (SA). (1989). SA Literature, P.O. Box 300, Simi Valley, CA.

Sex and Love Addicts Anonymous (SLAA). (1986). *Types of love and sex addiction.* Retrieved March 7, 2009, from http://www.slaafws.org/

LESSON 9 APPENDIX

Sexual Symptoms in Recovery Worksheet

The following questionnaire is aimed at evaluating problematic sexual behaviors *during the past 7 days*. Please read the questions carefully before you answer. Write a short description of the problematic sexual behavior you are evaluating:

_____

_____

Sexual health in recovery is taking the time to assess patterns of sexual behavior that continue despite placing your recovery at high risk.

1. If you had urges to engage in problematic sexual behaviors, on average, how strong were your urges to drink and use? Please circle the most appropriate number.

None	Mild	Moderate	Severe	Extreme
0	1	2	3	4

2. How many times did you experience urges to engage in problematic sexual behaviors? Please circle the most appropriate number.

None	Once	Two to three times	Several to many	Constant to near constant
0	1	2	3	4

3. How many hours (add up hours) were you preoccupied with your urges to engage in problematic sexual behaviors? Please circle the most appropriate number.

None	1 or less	1 to 7	7 to 21	More than 21
0	1	2	3	4

4. How much were you able to control your urges? Please circle the most appropriate number.

Completely	Much	Moderate	Minimal	No control
0	1	2	3	4

5. How often did thoughts about engaging in problematic sexual behaviors come up? Please circle the most appropriate number.

None	Once	Two to three times	Several to many	Constant to near constant
0	1	2	3	4

6. Approximately how many hours (add up hours) did you spend thinking about engaging in problematic sexual behaviors? Please circle the most appropriate number.

None	1 or less	1 to 7	7 to 21	More than 21
0	1	2	3	4

7. How much were you able to control your thoughts of problematic sexual behaviors to prevent using or drinking? Please circle the most appropriate number.

Completely	Much	Moderate	Minimal	No control
0	1	2	3	4

8. Approximately how much total time did you spend engaging in problematic sexual behaviors? Please circle the most appropriate number.

None	1 or less	1 to 7	7 to 21	More than 21
0	1	2	3	4

9. On average, how much anticipatory tension and/or excitement did you have *shortly before* you engaged in problematic sexual behaviors? If you did not actually engage in such behaviors, please estimate how much tension and/or excitement you believe you would have experienced if you had engaged in problematic sexual behaviors. Please circle the most appropriate number.

None	Mild	Moderate	Severe	Extreme
0	1	2	3	4

10. On average, how much excitement and pleasure did you feel when you engaged in problematic sexual behaviors? If you did not actually engage in such behaviors, please estimate how much excitement and pleasure you would have experienced, if you had. Please circle the most appropriate number.

None	Mild	Moderate	Severe	Extreme
0	1	2	3	4

11. How much emotional distress (stress, anguish, shame, guilt, embarrassment) has your problematic sexual behavior caused you? Please circle the most appropriate number.

None	Mild	Moderate	Severe	Extreme
0	1	2	3	4

12. How much risk of relapse (thoughts of using drugs or drinking, secretly planning to get high and have sex, using drugs, drinking) has your problematic sexual behavior caused you? Please circle the most appropriate number.

None	Mild	Moderate	Severe	Extreme
0	1	2	3	4

Adapted from Raymond, Lloyd, Miner, and Kim (2007); SSAS, Program in Human Sexuality, University of Minnesota.

Sexual Health

10

Sexual Functioning in Recovery

CORE CONCEPT

Sexual functioning in drug and alcohol recovery is an important (and often overlooked) component of relapse prevention. Addicts are in good company with the vast majority of Americans who lack basic knowledge and up-to-date sex research about why our sexual response functions or does not fully function. For addicts who may have used drugs or alcohol as a homemade remedy for sexual performance, this ignorance is a serious risk for relapse. A basic principle of sexual health in recovery is for women and men to understand their sexual functioning as a vital tool for staying sober.

In this session, participants will learn a newly emerging theory of sexual response. This dual control model for sexual response provides promising relapse prevention tools for men and women with sex/drug-linked concerns or worries about their sexual functioning. Experiential and interactive learning will provide a forum for candid and respectful discussion of sexual functioning. Men's and women's group discussion will focus on linking sexual arousal and sexual inhibition with drugs and alcohol as a dangerous solution for regulating these two components of sexual functioning. The "Sexual Health Recovery Scale for Women" and "Sexual Health Recovery scale for Men" are the relapse

241

prevention steps to stay aware, conscious, and intentional in actively addressing individual sexual response as a long-term recovery process.

BELIEF STATEMENT

Sexual health in recovery is the ability to understand sexual functioning in recovery.

OBJECTIVES

Participants will
- Learn the dual control model of sexual response.
- Increase awareness of how drug or alcohol use was an attempt to change sexual functioning.
- Think about sexual health attitudes and behaviors that increase sexual functioning in recovery.

CHANGE GOALS

- Understand how sexual functioning is a balance between feelings of sexual excitement and worries about sexual performance and negative consequences of sex.
- Incorporate sexual excitement and sexual inhibitors that support healthy sexual functioning in recovery.
- Utilize the "Sexual Health Recovery Scale for Women" and "Sexual Health Recovery scale for Men" to track relapse risk associated with sexual functioning.

REQUIRED READING FOR GROUP LEADER

New research on human sexual response provides an exciting opportunity for linking sex/drug-linked relapse risk with management of worries, problems, and disorders related to sexual functioning. Group leaders need to become familiar with the dual control model of sexual response (Bancroft, Graham, Janssen, & Sanders, 2009). The dual control theory proposes that both female and male sexual excitation and sexual inhibition combine to create an individual propensity for responding sexually. When sexual response is seen as an outcome stemming from the balance between brain excitation mechanisms and brain inhibition mechanisms a useful theory for understanding sex/drug-linked behavior emerges. Some drugs and alcohol reduce inhibitions. Other drugs increase excitation. Combing drugs and alcohol may do both. Understanding the dual control model for sexual response is an excellent fit for conceptualizing sex/drug-linked behavior. Providing recovering women and men a personal map for their sexual excitation and sexual inhibition may reduce sex/drug relapse risk. Shame resulting from sex and drug history may reduce when part of the sex/drug link seen as a misguided attempt to address concerns related to sexual functioning, sexual desire, or sexual response.

Inventories that measure male and female sexual excitement and sexual inhibition show a wide range of diversity in both genders. Men tend to score higher on excitation and lower on inhibition than women. Women with higher levels of excitement tended to take more sexual risks whereas sexual risk taking in men was more related to low inhibitions.

This lesson expands on the dual control theory by suggesting that a strong motivation for sex/drug-linked behavior is to adjust the balance between excitation and inhibition to better balance sexual arousal and therefore sexual response and functioning.

Sex/drug-linked behavior is an important behavioral component of managing sexual response for many using addicts. Some drugs increase arousal, sustain arousal, or allow for prolonged arousal. Other drugs decrease inhibitions, lesson inhibitions, or (in the extreme) eliminate inhibition via unconsciousness or blackout.

This lesson looks at how specific sex/drug-linked behaviors connect with two distinct sexual inhibitors. Each inhibitor is a kind of threat in the presence of sexual excitement. One threat is decreased sexual performance; the other threat is the anticipated consequence of sex. Some addicts may use specific drugs to eliminate the threat of decreased sexual performance, while others may continue to use drugs to avoid the negative consequences of the sex and pave the way for prolonged or uninterrupted sexual excitement.

RECOMMENDED MATERIALS FOR GROUP LEADER

- *Women's Sexualities* by Carol Ellison (Ellison, 2000) draws on the experiences of over 2,600 women to deepen knowledge about sexual development, partnered sex, and erotic pleasures. Her findings about women's experiences with fantasy, masturbation, sexual satisfaction, and orgasm (pp. 181–291) are excellent background material for leading both the women's and men's group. Ellison describes the complex and deeply meaningful world of a woman's arousal. Contrast women's arousal and inhibitor influences with the more straightforward influences on the male sexual response system. This will bring empathy and compassion toward group members as they reflect on the intricate balance of their individual sexual response through stories and examples.

■ *The Great Lover Playbook,* by international author and sex expert Lou Paget (2005), lists one sex tip for 365 days a year to keep sex alive and exciting for couples (same sex or opposite sex) who have been together for just a few week or decades. It is a good tool for group leaders to be familiar with quick answers to group members looking for detailed, specific sexual ideas for increasing arousal or decreasing inhibitors without relying on drugs or alcohol. Paget is a sex-positive sexologist who provides group leaders with examples of healthy language for engaging in lively group discussion.

■ Sex Smart Films (www.sexsmartfilms.com) is a Web-based film viewing and distribution site providing accurate sexual health information for adults of all ages. Every film on this site is an educational film. Sex Smart Films is an opportunity for group leaders to watch and learn from classic and contemporary sex educators, researchers, and therapists. An essential learning experience for counselors leading sexual health groups is to experience explicit sexual training materials with adult men and women having sex alone or with partners. Sex educators and therapists are unwavering in their recommendation of sexually explicit professionally produced training materials as basic training for all sex counselors. *Advanced Sexual Techniques and Positions,* produced by expert director and producer Mark Schoen, PhD, is a comprehensive review of male and female anatomy, sexual response, and orgasm as well as all stages of sexual activity from foreplay to oral sex, and a variety of sexual intercourse positions (Schoen, 2005). All examples are heterosexual couples. (Training materials with same-sex couples are available at Sex Smart Films.) An important bonus feature is listening to world renowned sex experts discussing their personal experiences with watching explicit sexual training films. They provide clear and compelling evidence that if a counselor is not comfortable with his or her own sexuality and the sexuality of others he or she will not be an effective educator or counselor. Sex training films are basic to expanding comfort with human sexuality as well as understanding the physical and embodied expression of the human sexual response.

REQUIRED MATERIALS FOR THE LESSON

- An mp3 player and music selection
- Blackboard, white board, or flip chart
- "How Much Am I Aroused?" (one copy for each participant) (Lesson 10 appendix, A)
- Set of building blocks
- "Sexual Health Recovery Scale for Men" (one copy for each male participant) (Lesson 10 appendix, B)
- "Sexual Health Recovery Scale for Women" (one copy for each female participant) (Lesson 10 appendix, C)

OPENING

Opening Music: *Have quiet music playing as participants enter the room and ready themselves (optional).*

Leader: As we sit quietly and focus on being here, let us clear our minds of where we have been and focus on being in this moment.

Opening Poem/Reading: Listen to this story told by a woman at an NA meeting:

When I left detox this was the first meeting I made. I sat up front and listened. Listening is a gift. It wasn't easy because my sick thinking was always working on me. I got a sponsor and a God of my understanding. In the beginning I only thought of getting with the men, but after being in the process for a little while, I noticed that the other women weren't doing this and I didn't have to either. I got some women in my life who gave me unconditional love and taught me how to wash everyday. I had a problem with hygiene: After so many years of not washing, I was uncomfortable that way. The women taught me how to be a lady, how to maintain good hygiene habits, and how to be loving and caring without sex.

—L. Green, M. Fullilove, and R. Fullilove,
"Remembering the Lizard" (2005)

GROUP INTRODUCTION

Have group member volunteer to read aloud.

Welcome to the sexual health in recovery group. We are here to talk about sex and how our sexual lives affect recovery from drug and alcohol addiction. Some people in recovery risk a relapse because of their sexual behavior at the treatment center or away from the treatment program. This is a place to talk about sexual behavior and sexual health so we can be abstinent from drugs and alcohol. It is also a place to learn about sexual behavior and situations that put men and women in recovery at risk for not completing this treatment program.

Sexual health in recovery is a time to talk about human sexuality and sexual health in a respectful and informed manner. We encourage everyone to be as honest and open as you can be. You are not required to reveal anything about your current or past sexual behavior that would be uncomfortable to discuss. It is important to listen to each other. For some of us, our sexual behavior is the most serious risk to staying in recovery. For others, our sexual behavior gets us into dangerous situations that are triggers to use or drink. A few of us may have little concern about how our sexual behavior contributes to relapse. This group is an opportunity for everyone to learn about the important connection between recovery and sexual health.

LESSON INTRODUCTION

Ask another group member to volunteer to read aloud.

The purpose of today's sexual behavior relapse prevention group is to learn important new information about the male and female sexual response. Sexual functioning is an important (and often overlooked) component of relapse prevention. For some recovering men and women, drugs and alcohol were a homemade remedy for concerns about their sexual performance. Without good information about human sexual response and a plan for addressing sexual functioning concerns, drug-addicted women and men are dangerously at risk for relapse. Women and men in recovery increase their likelihood of staying sober when they understand their sexual functioning in recovery.

Today we will learn an important new model of human sexual response that has important solutions for preventing relapse. We will learn that what turns us on and what puts the brakes on our arousal is a delicate balance that is specific to each person in this room. We will discuss together and in separate groups for men and women how drinking and using may have been a failed attempt to address concerns and worries about sexual functioning. We will learn how to use a sexual health assessment tool to actively assess sexual response as a long-term recovery tool.

LECTURE

Leader: Today we are going to learn a new model for understanding the sexual functioning of women and men. Men and women in recovery need to learn how to evaluate and enjoy their sexual signals in recovery while maintaining their abstinence from drugs and alcohol. Most of us do not realize that our sexual response system is actually quite fragile and can easily break down from using or abusing alcohol and drugs. We may have used drinking and drugs to change our sexual response. Recovery may lead us to new experiences and sensations in our sexual sparks and attractions. Some of these responses we have never before felt or sensed. Today, we are going to give you a new map for understanding the sexual responses of men and women. We will learn how to use this knowledge of sexual response as a relapse prevention tool.

First, let's review a little history. Did you know that most of the information we have about the human sexual response cycle has only been available for less than 40 years? Considering how long people have worried about their sexual functioning, it is quite amazing that chances are that your own parents and grandparents did not learn when they were your age what we are going to tell you. Some of you may have had sex education classes or opportunities to learn about the human sexual response. How many here have had a sex education class that explained the human sexual response?

Have participants raise their hands, invite any feedback about their previous learning experiences.

Leader: William Masters and Virginia Johnson were pioneering sex researchers who for the first time observed and measured sexual arousal in laboratory observations with adults who volunteered to be studied. It was the loosening of sexual boundaries that began in the mid 1960s that allowed this important scientific study to occur. Many other researchers have studied the human sexual response. You were probably taught a model that was fairly simple and straightforward. Until recently, sexual response was thought to be about the same between men and women. It was also thought to be a one-way path from desire, arousal, to really close to orgasm, orgasm, and then a period of waiting again for it to all be able to happen again. That period is much shorter for women; in fact, it may be so short that women can have several orgasms very close together. Men have a longer refractory period. This is different for different men and can change over time. Over the last 10 years, newer models of sexual response have been studied. We now know that these early sexual response models needed lots of improving.

We are going to learn one of the newest models for looking at our sexual response. The Kinsey Institute for Research in Sex, Gender and Reproduction, a world leader in sex research, proposes that our sexual functioning depends on the balance between sexual excitation and the forces that inhibit sexual function and response. Think of our sexual functioning like a moving car. A car can speed up or slow down. We can slow our car down by either taking our foot off the gas pedal or by putting our foot on the brake. These two pedals work independently and yet are linked in that they both influence how the car behaves. The dual control model of sexual response works in a similar manner. What excites us sexually speeds us up, arouses us, turns us on, and gets us hot. This is our gas pedal. We can have a less excited car by just not pressing the gas pedal so far down. We don't even have to touch the brake. Easing up on the gas, the car will slow down.

This new sex research is leading us to believe that everyone has a general range of excitement and arousal. In other words, some of us have the ability for high sexual arousal. Others have a relatively low range for arousal. These are normal differences and we now believe there is a wide range in the way men and women typically become sexually aroused and excited. What results in sexual arousal varies from person to person so much that we cannot say there is a correct or perfect way to become sexually excited. What is more important for sexual health in recovery is to learn about your own personal sexual response: both what excites you and what inhibits you.

The central assumption of the dual control model (Bancroft et al., 2009) is that sexual arousal and response result from a balance between inhibitory and excitatory mechanisms of the central nervous system. This balance between sexual excitement and sexual inhibition is like a balancing act between two different forces in the brain. This interaction between arousal and suppression is very different among many people. There is not a correct way to experience this interaction. The dual control model assumes that most people can adjust their sexual inhibitions because of the environment, situation, or circumstances in the moment. It is this adjustment, the brakes of our sexual response, that is necessary for us to avoid sexually risky or threatening situations. If we have too strong brakes or not strong enough brakes, meaning our inhibition levels are either constantly too low or too high, this contributes to problems ranging from high-risk sexual behavior (not enough brakes to balance the arousal) to sexual dysfunctions such as no desire for sex or erection and orgasm problems (too much brake and not enough arousal to balance out the brake). This would be like trying to leave a parking spot and keeping the parking brake on and only driving the car in first gear.

So, in sexual terms, when strong sexual inhibition is paired with low sexual excitation, sexual response may be particularly impaired. You are just not going to be turned on very much if at all. On the other side, if low sexual inhibition is combined with high excitation, you have little stopping your level of arousal and may move quickly and easily towards high-risk sexual situations. When we are highly sexually aroused we usually do not always think as clearly. Adding drugs or alcohol to an already speeding sexual arousal may lead to sexual risk-taking. Sexual risk-taking behavior and sexual functioning problems are sexual health in recovery issues of significant personal and social concern for everyone in recovery. This dual control model of sexual response provides a working concept and set of ideas to outline our human sexual response. Most importantly, it shows how drugs and alcohol may link with our sexual response system. Understanding our individual sexual excitement and inhibition responses may reduce the risk of sex/drug-linked relapse risk.

If a woman in recovery knows she is a high arouser and has used certain drugs to increase her inhibitions so she doesn't have sex so quickly, she will need to establish ways to live with her likely tendency of high arousal and discover inhibitors that are not drugs or alcohol. If a man is an average arouser, he will need to either decrease or increase his inhibitors in specific sexual situations so he can feel aroused and excited. Of course he will need to experiment with ways to regulate his inhibitors without resorting to drugs and alcohol. A better understanding of these differences in arousal and inhibition may potentially improve sexual problems and sex/drug-linked behavior risks in recovery.

The good news is we don't just have to ease up on our arousal to have responsible and pleasurable sex. We also have a brake pedal. We will talk about the sexual brake pedal later. For now we just want to have you understand that for men and women their sexual response is an individual dance between excitation and inhibition, acceleration and braking.

Our sexual functioning is a unique personal recipe, some of which may be genetic, situational, cultural, and of course mental (in our brains). Drugs and alcohol significantly alter both sexual excitement and sexual suppression. Sexual health in recovery is the process of learning our sexual functioning. Men and women in recovery need to learn what is sexually exciting and arousing as well as understand what inhibitions balance out his or her arousal.

EXPERIENTIAL LEARNING

Leader: Let's look at a variety of sexual situations, behaviors, or situations. We are going privately and individually measure or rate whether the statement is describing something that is exciting, arousing, or a turn on.

Hand out "How Much Am I Aroused?" (Lesson 10 appendix, A), which contains 16 items, each with a rating scale of one through five.

Leader: As I read each statement, I want you to quickly choose a number one to five. The higher the number, the more you agree that the statement would be arousing. The lower the number, the less you agree. Try to be as honest as possible. There are no right or wrong answers. Don't think too long. If it does not apply to you, then rate what you would choose if you thought it did apply to you. Of course your answer would vary depending on the circumstance, but for this exercise, just answer based on what would be your most likely reaction.

Do a practice item from the scale. (Use the first item, "I read something sexual in a book.") Then go through all the items.

Leader: Now we will go over these again, but this time the situation is that you have been using, drinking, or both.

Go through the list again. Circle the rating of agreement to disagreement on the second list of Lesson 10 appendix, A—"How Much Am I Aroused After Drinking or Using Drugs?" Lead a discussion of what people noticed was different in their ratings of arousal/excitement when using/drinking as opposed to when sober.

Leader: What is important to know about this? Did being high make you more or less turned on? Did what you were using make a difference?

Lead a discussion about which drugs made for less arousal and more arousal.

Leader: Excitation or lack of excitation is not enough to describe our sexual response. Feelings of sexual excitement, feeling horny, hot, or turned on or the lack of this feeling is not enough to understand sexual response or functioning. What is a turn on for one person in one situation may not be exciting in another. Why is this? Something must be balancing out the excitement. Remember our car brake pedal? In addition to having low, medium, or high arousal we can also have different levels of sexual response if the brake is pushed softly, firmly, or very hard. Just like going real fast in a car, our arousal can accelerate really fast. Without brakes, just taking our foot off the gas won't slow the car down in enough time to avoid a terrible outcome. The Kinsey Institute has found that the brakes for women and the brakes for men are different. What inhibits sexual arousal for men and for women have some important differences. We will now divide into our men's and women's groups to discuss these sex differences.

Break into separate groups of men and women. Both groups will meet for the remainder of the session in separate private rooms, each with at least one group leader.

MEN'S GROUP

Leader: As we get comfortable in our group of just men, I want to start out by reviewing what we will do with the remainder of our time. We will spend some of the time in general discussion about sexual inhibitors. We will end the group with some practice time to learn how to use the "Sexual Health Recovery Scale for Men."

The first important part of this model for sexual response is that it is just like a car. Cars actually have two brake systems. One is the brake pedal, and the other is the emergency brake. We use the emergency brake when the car is parked to keep it from moving without someone driving. We use the brake pedal for driving. In an extreme emergency, when our brake pedal is not working, we use the emergency brake to stop us from real danger or injury. Our sexual inhibitors work the same way. And just like a car, this system works best and most safely when the driver is sober.

The Kinsey Institute was surprised to discover a two-brake system for sexual inhibitions. The two inhibitors balance our sexual arousal with a threat. In other words, sexual arousal will always feel good and be pretty intensely interesting to pursue, just like going fast in a car usually feels good. Part of the reason it feels good to go fast is that we have brakes we trust, that will work when we need them. This is how a threat works to balance the thrill of arousal. The brakes on a moving car are like our sexual inhibitors. Sexual inhibitions are very important. They help avoid sexually risky or threatening situations. Inhibitors can be danger, a risk, potential harm, or a really negative consequence, especially if it leads to shame or embarrassment. Of most importance for the men in this room is the additional risk of using or drinking. Sexual health in recovery is about making sure we respect our inhibitors so they keep us from avoiding sex/drug-linked situations in which we are not able to manage the arousal.

The Kinsey Institute researchers found two types of threats (brake pedal and emergency brake) that inhibit our sexual excitement. One is a threat related to sexual performance. For men, anticipating loss of sexual arousal is a big concern. If a man thinks or anticipates not performing sexually, it will turn the heat down pretty fast. The threat of not performing sexually is the brake pedal. What are some common sexual performance threats that men worry about?

> *Listen for themes in each group member's statement. Reflect back to group members if their example fits with a worry of not getting or not maintaining an erection, not pleasing their partners, or being distracted by other thoughts or concern and rapid ejaculation. How might drugs or alcohol have been an attempt to remedy these concerns?*

Leader: The second set of inhibitors has to do with unpleasant consequences of having sex or after the sex is complete. This is the equivalent of using your car brake because you see cars on the road ahead of you slowing down, or you know the road may be icy or slippery ahead. This is when we can see ahead just a few seconds to months or even years later and put on the brakes because we do not want the consequence that we have reasoned may result from having sex. What consequences can happen during or after sex (not related to sexual performance) that come to mind? How has drinking or using been related to these consequences? What are some really embarrassing, humiliating, painful, scary, or just unpleasant consequences?

Lead a discussion about embarrassing, humiliating, painful, scary, or just unpleasant consequences of having sex that men may experience. Remind the group it is not necessary to share personal experience; the group is not a therapy group for sharing personal stories that we do not have the time to attend to in the lesson. We are interested in sharing ideas.

Leader: Women tend to be more inhibited (put the brakes on) toward having sex when feeling emotionally disconnected with their partners. Men do not put on the brakes as much when emotionally disconnected with their partners. In early recovery, women may focus on relationships as a means of learning about their sexual arousal because they have much less sexual excitement without the context of a relationship. Men in early recovery may be less focused on relational sex, partly because men tend be much more capable of sexual excitement in casual sex and one night stands. Men may learn a great deal about their sexual inhibitions in early recovery through solo sex. Masturbation is a very important way to explore excitement and sexual inhibitions in early recovery. How might risk of relapse be a factor in men who can become easily sexually excited in a casual, nonrelational situation?

Lead a discussion, again without an emphasis on personal disclosure, but rather with discussion focused on the many ways men can be sexually excited in situations that women tend to not be as readily excited. For gay identified men or men who have sex with men, this is an especially important discussion. Having two men in the sexual situation has a multiple effect of having both sexual partners with the same ability to be more readily aroused in a nonrelational situation. Emphasize this magnification of arousal and minimization of inhibitors when both partners are men.

Topic Skill Practice

Take out building blocks for demonstration. Have at least five different stacks of blocks.

Leader: Let's demonstrate what this sexual response system looks like by using a set of building blocks. Each building block is either an inhibitor or an arouser. Each block therefore represents sexual excitement, a threat of sexual performance or a threat of a negative consequence either during or after sex. Each man has his own individual stable level of inhibition, meaning that when a man is in a state of no sexual arousal and excitement he has a set level of built-in inhibitors.

Place one block on the table to demonstrate the set level of built-in inhibitors a man has in a state of no sexual arousal.

Leader: Some men may have a high level of a set state of sexual inhibition.

Place four blocks on the table to demonstrate a higher state of built-in inhibitors for some men in a state of no sexual arousal.

Leader: In order to have sufficient arousal to balance the steady set amount of inhibitors, you need enough arousal to balance this.

Build an arousal stack of blocks and an inhibitor stack. The arousal stack should be just a bit higher than the inhibitor stack.

Leader: Remember the list of arousers we discussed in the large group? If you have high inhibitors, you need high arousal to experience full sexual functioning. Sexual researchers have found that individuals who score highly in inhibition might be more likely to experience sexual problems. Men with high sexual inhibition may focus on decreasing the inhibitor level so the level of arousal is enough to sexually function.

Demonstrate this idea by removing a few blocks from the inhibitor stack so it is much lower than the arousal blocks. Have the group discuss various ways addicts and alcoholics use drinking and drugs to change this balance.

Leader: Now let's look at the reverse situation. A man may have very low level of inhibitors as his set point. He may have an ability to feel highly sexually aroused when completely sober.

Using the building blocks, place a very high stack of arousers next to small stack of inhibitors.

Leader: What are the possible problems this man may confront in recovery?

Lead a brief discussion about possible behaviors and situations a man in recovery may find himself in if he has this imbalance.

Leader: This is why we developed the "Sexual Health Recovery Scale for Men." It is a tool to evaluate your current frequency of actions, attitudes, and sexual behaviors that support a more balanced healthy sexual functioning between your arousers and inhibitors. The higher the score, the less likely your sexual response or sexual function will be a relapse risk.

Hand out the "Sexual Health Recovery Scale for Men" (Lesson 10 appendix, B) and review how to fill out the form. Have group members complete the form before ending group. Encourage members to discuss their scores with their sexual recovery support teams.

Leader: You all did a great job with this exercise and with talking about sexual functioning and sexual response. I will hand out blank copies of this worksheet for you to take with you. Make copies of this for future use. See how your scores change over the next 12 months.

Closing

Leader: Now let's take a moment to bring the workshop to a close. Lets take a moment to again quiet ourselves, take a deep breath to quiet our minds, our hearts, and our spirits. In this quiet place, remind yourself how valuable it is to take the time to learn about our sexual functioning and how the experiences of sexual desire, arousal, and orgasm play a role in every recovering addict's sobriety and well-being. As you leave the group today, remind yourself that a satisfying sexual life is a vital and important part of recovery. The sexual functioning information and the sexual functioning recovery scale may become important parts of maintaining your recovery.

WOMEN'S GROUP

Leader: As we get comfortable in our group of women, I want to start out by reviewing what we will do with the remainder of our time. We will spend some of the time in general discussion about sexual inhibitors. We will end the group with some practice time to learn how to use the "Sexual Health Recovery Scale for Women."

The first important part of this model for sexual response is that it is just like a car. Cars actually have two brake systems. One is the brake pedal, and the other is the emergency brake. We use the emergency brake when the car is parked to keep it from moving without someone driving. We use the brake pedal for driving. In an extreme emergency, when our brake pedal is not working, we use the emergency brake to stop us from real danger or injury. Our sexual inhibitors work the same way. And just like a car this system works best and most safely when the driver is sober.

The Kinsey Institute was surprised to discover a two-brake system for sexual inhibitions. The two inhibitors balance our sexual arousal with a threat. In other words, sexual arousal will always feel good and be pretty intensely interesting to pursue, just like going fast in a car usually feels good. Part of the reason it feels good to go fast is that we have brakes we trust, that will work when we need them. This is how a threat works to balance the thrill of arousal. The brakes on a moving car are like our sexual inhibitors. Sexual inhibitions are very important. They help avoid sexually risky or threatening situations. Inhibitors can be danger, a risk, potential harm, or a really negative consequence, especially if it leads to shame or embarrassment. Of most importance for the women in this room is the additional risk of using or drinking. Sexual health in recovery is about making sure we respect our inhibitors so they keep us from avoiding sex/drug-linked situations in which we are not able to manage the arousal.

The Kinsey Institute researchers found two types of threats that inhibit our sexual excitement. One is a threat related to sexual performance. For women, anticipating difficulty getting aroused or losing arousal because of distractions is a common concern. If a woman anticipates not feeling sexually interested or excited, it will turn the heat down pretty fast. (See "The Sexual Excitation/Sexual Inhibition Inventory for Women," pp. 125–126 and Appendix B, pp. 141–142 in Bancroft et al., 2009). The threat of difficulty becoming aroused is the brake pedal. What are some common sexual performance threats that women worry about?

> *Listen for themes in each group member's statement. Reflect back to group members how their examples fit with a worry of arousal being disrupted by concerns about pregnancy, body image, weight, mood, stress, sexual setting, and sexual partner attributes. How might drugs or alcohol have been an attempt to remedy these concerns?*

Leader: The second set of inhibitors has to do with unpleasant consequences of having sex or after the sex is complete. This is the equivalent of using your car brake because you see cars on the road ahead of you slowing down, or you know the road may be icy or slippery ahead. This is when we can see ahead just a few seconds to months or even years later and put on the brakes because we do not want the consequence that we have reasoned may result from having sex. What consequences can happen during or after sex (not related to sexual performance) that come to mind? How has drinking or using been related to these consequences? What are some really embarrassing, humiliating, painful, lifelong, or just unpleasant consequences?

Lead a discussion about embarrassing, humiliating , painful, lifelong, or just unpleasant consequences of having sex that women may experience. Remind the group it is not necessary to share personal experience; the group is not a therapy group for sharing personal stories that we do not have the time to attend to in the lesson. We are interested in sharing ideas.

Leader: What consequences can happen during or after sex (not related to sexual performance) that come to mind? What are some really embarrassing, humiliating, painful, lifelong or just unpleasant consequences?

Listen for women worrying about the impact of sex on their reputation, feeling distant, angry, physically unsafe, emotionally unsafe, insufficient privacy, nonconsensual sex, feeling undesired, feeling exploited, used, objectified, acquiring a sexually transmitted infection, religion, femininity, being improper, and being thought of as "too loose." How has drinking or using been related to these consequences?

Topic Skill Practice

Take out building blocks for demonstration. Have at least five different stacks of blocks.

Leader: Let's demonstrate what this sexual response system looks like by using a set of building blocks. Each building block is either an inhibitor or an arouser. Each block therefore represents sexual excitement, a threat of sexual performance or a threat of a negative consequence either during or after sex. Each woman has her own individual stable level of inhibition, meaning that when a woman is in a state of no sexual arousal and excitement she has a set level of built-in inhibitors.

Place one block on table to demonstrate the set level of built-in inhibitors a woman has in a state of no sexual arousal.

Leader: Some women may have a high level of a set state of sexual inhibition.

Place four blocks on the table to demonstrate a higher state of built-in inhibitors for some women in a state of no sexual arousal.

Leader: In order to have sufficient arousal to balance the steady set amount of inhibitors, a woman will need enough arousal to balance this high level of inhibitions.

Build an arousal stack of blocks and an inhibitor stack. The arousal stack should be just a bit higher than the inhibitor stack.

Leader: Remember the list of arousers we discussed in the large group. Women with high inhibitors, may need high and uninterrupted arousal to experience full sexual functioning. Preliminary Sex research on the dual control model for women suggests a much more complex picture of sexual problems related to desire, arousal, and climax (see pp. 133–134 in Bancroft et al., 2009). Women in one sex research study who reported the strongest predictor of sexual problems were women with high frequency of needing things just right or they were easily turned off and had difficulty staying aroused (Sanders, Graham, & Milhausen, 2008). For women, much more research is needed to understand the relationship between excitation and inhibition.

Demonstrate this idea by asking group members to identify an inhibitor that interferes with arousal. Remove a few blocks from the inhibitor stack when a woman in the group thinks that if that particular inhibitor was not present she could focus more on her arousal.

Have the group discuss various ways women with addictions and alcoholism use drinking and drugs to change this balance between arousal and inhibition.

Leader: Now let's look at the reverse situation. A woman may have a very low level of inhibitors as her set point. She may have an ability to feel highly sexually aroused when completely sober.

Using the blocks, place a very high stack of arousers next to small stack of inhibitors.

Leader: What are the possible problems this woman may confront in recovery?

Lead a brief discussion about possible behaviors and situations a woman in recovery may find herself in with this imbalance.

Leader: This is why we developed the "Sexual Health Recovery Scale for Women." It is a tool to evaluate your current frequency of actions, attitudes, and sexual behaviors that support a healthy sexual functioning. The higher the score, the less likely your sexual response or sexual function will be a relapse risk.

Hand out the "Sexual Health Recovery Scale for Women" (Lesson 10 appendix, C) and review how to fill out the form. Have group members complete the form before ending group. Encourage members to discuss their scores with their sexual recovery support teams.

Leader: You all did a great job with this exercise and with talking about sexual functioning and sexual response. I will hand out blank copies of this worksheet for you to take with you. Make copies of this for future use. See how your scores change over the next 12 months.

Closing

Leader: Now let's take a moment to bring the workshop to a close. Let's take a moment to again quiet ourselves, take a deep breath to quiet our minds, our hearts, and our spirits. In this quiet place, remind yourself how valuable it is to take the time to learn about our sexual functioning and how the experiences of sexual desire, arousal, and orgasm play a role in every recovering addict's sobriety and well-being. As you leave the group today, remind yourself that a satisfying sexual life is a vital and important part of recovery. The sexual functioning information and the sexual functioning recovery scale may become important parts of maintaining your recovery.

REFERENCES

Bancroft, J., Graham, C., Janssen, E., & Sanders, S. (2009). The dual control model: Current status and future directions. *Journal of Sex Research, 46*(2-3), 121–142.

Ellison, C. (2000). *Women's sexualities.* The Read File Publishing Company.

Green, L., Fullilove, M., & Fullilove, R., (2005). Remembering the lizard: Reconstructing sexuality in the rooms of narcotics anonymous. *The Journal of Sex Research, 42*(1), 28–34.

Paget, L. (2005). The great lover playbook. New York: Gotham Books.

Sanders, S., Graham, C., & Milhausen, R. (2008). Predicting sexual problems in women: The relevance of sexual excitation and sexual inhibition. *Archives of Sexual Behavior, 37*, 241–251.

Schoen, M. (Producer). (2005). *Advanced sexual techniques and positions* [Motion picture]. United States: Sinclair Intimacy Institute.

Sex Smart Films. (2009). Retrieved from www.SexSmartFilms.com

LESSON 10 APPENDIX

A. How Much Am I Aroused?

As you hear each item read aloud circle the number that reflects how much you agree that the situation or description is typically sexually arousing for you. If you have not been in the situation, imagine how arousing you think it may be for you and then answer the question. There are no right or wrong answers. (This list is adapted from Bancroft et al., 2009.)

How Much Am I Aroused?
1. I read something sexual in a book.
2. A sexually attractive stranger looks me in the eye.
3. I talk to someone on the phone with a sexy voice.
4. I have a quiet candlelight dinner with someone I find sexually attractive.
5. An attractive person flirts with me online.
6. I see someone I find attractive dressed in a sexy way.
7. Someone sexually attractive wants to have sex with me.
8. A sexually attractive stranger accidentally touches me.
9. I see others engaged in sex.
10. I am with a group of people watching a sex video online or on TV.
11. I am alone watching a sexual scene in a film.
12. I start fantasizing about sex.
13. I think about a sexual encounter I have had.
14. I look at erotic pictures.
15. I wear something I feel attractive in.
16. Someone sexually attractive is high and wants to have sex with me.

1. Strongly agree   Agree   Disagree   Strongly disagree
2. Strongly agree   Agree   Disagree   Strongly disagree
3. Strongly agree   Agree   Disagree   Strongly disagree
4. Strongly agree   Agree   Disagree   Strongly disagree
5. Strongly agree   Agree   Disagree   Strongly disagree
6. Strongly agree   Agree   Disagree   Strongly disagree
7. Strongly agree   Agree   Disagree   Strongly disagree
8. Strongly agree   Agree   Disagree   Strongly disagree
9. Strongly agree   Agree   Disagree   Strongly disagree
10. Strongly agree   Agree   Disagree   Strongly disagree

11. Strongly agree   Agree   Disagree   Strongly disagree
12. Strongly agree   Agree   Disagree   Strongly disagree
13. Strongly agree   Agree   Disagree   Strongly disagree
14. Strongly agree   Agree   Disagree   Strongly disagree
15. Strongly agree   Agree   Disagree   Strongly disagree
16. Strongly agree   Agree   Disagree   Strongly disagree

Total score_____

How Much Am I Aroused After Drinking or Using Drugs?

As you hear each item read aloud, circle the number that reflects how much you agree that the situation or description is typically sexually arousing for you when you have been drinking and/or using drugs. If you have not been in the situation, imagine how arousing you think it may be for you and then answer the question. There are no right or wrong answers.

1. Strongly agree   Agree   Disagree   Strongly disagree
2. Strongly agree   Agree   Disagree   Strongly disagree
3. Strongly agree   Agree   Disagree   Strongly disagree
4. Strongly agree   Agree   Disagree   Strongly disagree
5. Strongly agree   Agree   Disagree   Strongly disagree
6. Strongly agree   Agree   Disagree   Strongly disagree
7. Strongly agree   Agree   Disagree   Strongly disagree
8. Strongly agree   Agree   Disagree   Strongly disagree
9. Strongly agree   Agree   Disagree   Strongly disagree
10. Strongly agree   Agree   Disagree   Strongly disagree
11. Strongly agree   Agree   Disagree   Strongly disagree
12. Strongly agree   Agree   Disagree   Strongly disagree
13. Strongly agree   Agree   Disagree   Strongly disagree
14. Strongly agree   Agree   Disagree   Strongly disagree
15. Strongly agree   Agree   Disagree   Strongly disagree
16. Strongly agree   Agree   Disagree   Strongly disagree

Total score_____

B. Sexual Health Recovery Scale for Men

This is a 30-item self-assessment checklist. Each item is a description of a sexual behavior, thought, or experience. Rate yourself on the frequency that you have experienced each situation in the last 3 months. The level of frequency of these sexual activities can improve your sexual functioning and increase your chances of maintaining your recovery

1 = Never; 2 = Seldom; 3 = Occasionally; 4 = Often; 5 = Repeatedly

_____I find sex pleasurable.

_____I talk about my sexuality with my doctor as it relates to health care.

_____I talk about my sexual functioning concerns with informed and knowledgeable persons.

_____I am able to keep my healthy sexual boundaries.

_____I fantasize about sex.

_____I have interest in having sex.

_____The sex I have had while sober is satisfying.

_____I feel free to be sexual without drugs or alcohol.

_____I have orgasms.

_____Having an orgasm is an important part of having sex.

_____I am unlikely to stay aroused during sex if there is a risk of unwanted pregnancy.

_____I can get or keep an erection.

_____I can control my arousal so I only orgasm when I am ready.

_____I stay erect when I put on a condom.

_____I like how I can wait to have an orgasm until I am ready.

_____I feel intimate and close with my partner during sex.

_____I feel relaxed and comfortable after having an orgasm.

_____My desires to have sex are an enjoyable part of my daily life.

_____I have an interest in specific sexual turn-ons.

_____My sexual behavior is compatible with my recovery program.

_____I enjoy sex when I am sober.

_____I feel more confident that my sexual behavior will not lead to a relapse.

_____I take responsibility for my sexual satisfaction and pleasure.

_____I take responsibility to communicate to my sex partners what I need sexually.

_____I enjoy masturbation.

_____I usually think ahead about the potential consequences for having sex.

_____I have not allowed myself to just not care about my sexual behavior.

_____I like how I feel intensely passionate when I have sex.

_____I stop my sexual behavior when my partner is hurt or feeling pain.

_____I am interested in learning more about how my body responds to sexual arousal.

_____ Total score

The highest possible score is 150. Any score above 90 is a fairly good sign that your sexual functioning is a strong support of your recovery. Scores of less than 60 may be an indication of sexual functioning as a risk factor in relapse. Review any item you rated less than 3 and circle the items that you think play a role in increasing your risk for relapse. Focus on at least one of the circled items in your next 3 months of recovery.

C. Sexual Health Recovery Scale for Women

This is a 31-item self-assessment checklist. Each item is a description of a sexual behavior, thought, or experience. Rate yourself on the frequency that you have experienced each situation in the last 3 months. The level of frequency of these sexual activities can improve your sexual functioning and increase your chances of maintaining your recovery

1 = Never; 2 = Seldom; 3 = Occasionally; 4 = Often; 5 = Repeatedly

_____I find sex pleasurable.

_____I talk about my sexuality with my doctor as it relates to health care.

_____I talk about my sexual functioning concerns with informed and knowledgeable people.

_____I am able to keep my healthy sexual boundaries.

_____I fantasize about sex.

_____I have interest in having sex.

_____The sex I have had while sober is satisfying.

_____I feel free to be sexual without drugs or alcohol.

_____I have orgasms.

_____Having an orgasm is an important part of having sex.

_____I am interested in sex.

_____I make sexual choices around the cycle of my period.

_____I can control my arousal so I only get off when I am ready.

_____I enjoy my partner paying attention to me when having sex.

_____I like how I can wait and have an orgasm when I am ready.

_____My genitals respond when I feel aroused.

_____I feel comfortable during sexual intercourse with a sex partner.

_____I enjoy having clitoral stimulation.

_____My desires to have sex are an enjoyable part of my daily life.

_____I have an interest in specific sexual turn-ons.

_____My sexual behavior is compatible with my recovery program.

_____I enjoy sex when I am sober.

_____I feel more confident that my sexual behavior will not lead to a relapse.

_____I take responsibility for my sexual satisfaction and pleasure.

_____I take responsibility to communicate to my sex partners what I need sexually.

_____I enjoy being sexually playful.

_____I enjoy being seductive.

_____I like how I feel when I have feelings of sexual desire.

_____I like how I feel intensely passionate when I have sex.

_____I stop having sex when I am hurt or feeling pain.

_____I am interested in learning more about how my body responds to sexual arousal.

_____Total score

The highest possible score is 150. Any score above 90 is a fairly good sign that your sexual functioning is a strong support of your recovery. Scores of less than 60 may be an indication of sexual functioning as a risk factor in relapse. Review any item you rated less than 3 and circle the items that you think play a role in increasing your risk for relapse. Focus on at least one the circled items in your next 3 months of recovery.

11

Sexual Boundaries in Recovery

CORE CONCEPT

Boundary concerns are a central component of sexual health in recovery. Sexual health boundaries provide safe, professional, and effective chemical dependency treatment. Having healthy and responsible sexual boundaries is essential for recovery from drug and alcohol addiction. The sexual behavior relapse prevention curriculum is focused on healthy sexual boundaries that will increase the likelihood of completing treatment as well as maintaining sobriety after completing treatment.

The session will start by defining boundaries and specifically sexual boundaries. We will learn that boundaries exist on a continuum from boundary challenges to boundary crossings to boundary violations (Gutheil & Brodsky, 2008). Experiential interactive exercises relevant to residential and outpatient drug treatment provide participants with opportunities for exploring sexual boundaries within a recovery program. This workshop includes "The Sexual Boundaries in Recovery Inventory" for self-reporting boundary choices within the three-phase continuum of boundary issues. The inventory will be an opportunity to measure risk of relapse related to sexual health boundaries.

BELIEF STATEMENT

Sexual health in recovery is the ability to develop and practice sexual boundaries that enhance and support recovery.

OBJECTIVES

Participants will
- Define the concepts of boundaries and sexual boundaries.
- Identify the purpose of sexual boundaries in drug and alcohol treatment and recovery.
- Discuss the continuum of sexual boundary regulation.
- Increase understanding of regulation of sexual boundaries and relapse prevention.
- Provide role-play and experiential exercises to rehearse and understand sexual boundaries in recovery.

CHANGE GOALS

- Increase awareness of risk factors for relapse connected with crossing sexual boundaries.
- Understand the continuum of sexual boundaries and the range of consequences of errors in sexual boundary judgments and decisions.
- Utilize "The Sexual Boundaries in Recovery Inventory."

REQUIRED READING FOR GROUP LEADER

- *Preventing Boundary Violations in Clinical Practice* (Gutheil & Brodsky, 2008) reviews a continuum of boundaries in the first chapter (see pp. 15–21) that is the basis for the experiential exercises in this lesson. The publication is for clinicians of any theoretical orientation to understand the principles of boundaries in a mental health care setting. It is very relevant for drug and alcohol treatment. This material is vital for bringing familiarity to the concepts and using the tone of the written material to assist in leading the experiential exercises.

- *Boundaries: A Guide for Teens* (Peter & Dowd, 2000) is a small notebook bound book from Boys Town Press. It is written for teens and is about teens and their navigation of boundaries. Chapter 3, "Unhealthy Boundaries" (pp. 35–46), was source material for part of the "Unhealthy Boundaries" handout for this lesson.
- *Boundaries: Where You End and I Begin,* by Anne Katherine (1993), was also source material for development of "The Sexual Boundaries in Recovery Inventory." This is a comprehensive review of a wide array of emotional and physical boundaries men and women face in day-to-day life. Katherine brings a practical, example-filled profile of multiple levels of boundary concerns with clear, concise directions for resolution. The book is an excellent resource for the leader to be familiar with for addressing multiple boundary concerns clients present in this lesson.

RECOMMENDED MATERIALS FOR GROUP LEADER

I recommend three resources for more in-depth exploration of the meaning and complexity of boundaries as they pertain to sexual health among men and women in recovery.

- Chapter 2 of Stephanie Covington's book *Awakening Your Sexuality: A Guide for Recovering Women* (Covington, 2000) is about the sexual lies that are present in the lives of recovering women that separate them from their inner selves. Covington describes the brutal consequences of this rigid boundary on the sexual lives of women in recovery. She observes "No one seems to be able to talk about sex or to want to try, and it's rarely discussed even in therapy. Yet, as we know, only when denial is examined and replaced with truth and understanding does change become possible" (Covington, 2000, p. 28). I find this prescient statement all the more disheartening when almost 20 years later (HarperCollins originally published *Awakening Your Sexuality* in 1991) sex/drug-linked behavior in drug and alcohol treatment remains in the margins.
- I strongly recommend Chapter 3 in *Consent to Sexual Relations* (Wertheimer, 2003). Alan Wertheimer articulately and with splendid detail describes the all-too-common boundary violations that result when people do not want to engage in sexual relations and

sex becomes an unwanted or aversive nonconsensual experience. Wertheimer helps the reader understand why boundary violations surrounding sexual consent have been a problem throughout human history and across cultures. He discusses the evolutionary psychology of sex to explain why women respond the way they do to the very serious boundary violations inherent in nonconsensual sex as well as to understand why (mostly) men violate the sexual consent boundary.

- Finally, *Boundaries: Stop Getting Abused and Learn Healthy Boundaries* (Wagner, 2006) is a 31-minute educational psychology DVD. In a fairly straightforward lecture format in a small classroom setting, Jeff Gazley describes boundaries, setting boundaries, and the benefits of self-protection from abuse. The lecture goes past typical boundary content by discussing how to defend healthy boundaries and minimize offending others in the process. A free preview is available online at http://www.asktheinternettherapist. com/psychology_videos.asp.

REQUIRED MATERIALS FOR THE LESSON

- An mp3 player and music selection
- Blackboard, white board, or flip chart
- "Unhealthy Boundaries" (one copy for each participant) (Lesson 11 appendix, A)
- "The Sexual Boundaries in Recovery Inventory" (one copy for each participant) (Lesson 11 appendix, B)

OPENING

Opening Music: *Have quiet music playing as participants enter the room and ready themselves (optional).*

Leader: As we sit quietly and focus on being here, let us clear our minds of where we have been and focus on being in this moment.

Opening Poem/Reading:

Boundaries bring order to our lives. As we learn to strengthen our boundaries, we gain a clearer sense of ourselves and our relationship to others.

Boundaries empower us to determine how we'll be treated by others. With good boundaries, we can have the wonderful assurance that comes from knowing we can and will protect ourselves from the ignorance, meanness, and thoughtlessness of others.

—A. Katherine, Boundaries (1993)

Autobiography in Five Short Chapters by Portia Nelson

Chapter One

> I walk down the street.
> There is a deep hole in the sidewalk.
> I fall in
> I am lost
> I am hopeless
> It isn't my fault.
> It takes forever to find a way out.

Chapter Two

> I walk down the same street,
> There is a deep hole in the sidewalk.
> I pretend I don't see it.
> I fall in again.
> I can't believe I am in the same place.
> But it isn't my fault.
> It still takes a long time to get out.

Chapter Three

> I walk down the same street
> There is a deep hole in the sidewalk.
> I see it there.
> I fall in . . .
> It's a habit.
> My eyes are open.
> I know where I am.
> It is my fault.
> I get out immediately.

Chapter Four

> I walk down the same street.
> There is a deep hole in the sidewalk.
> I walk around it.

Chapter Five
   I walk down another street.

                              —Portia Nelson, *There's a Hole in My Sidewalk* (1993)

GROUP INTRODUCTION

Have group member volunteer to read aloud.
   Welcome to the sexual health in recovery group. We are here to talk about sex and how our sexual lives affect recovery from drug and alcohol addiction. Some people in recovery risk a relapse because of their sexual behavior at the treatment center or away from the treatment program. This is a place to talk about sexual behavior and sexual health so we can be abstinent from drugs and alcohol. It is also a place to learn about sexual behavior and situations that put men and women in recovery at risk for not completing this treatment program.
   Sexual health in recovery is a time to talk about human sexuality and sexual health in a respectful and informed manner. We encourage everyone to be as honest and open as you can be. You are not required to reveal anything about your current or past sexual behavior that would be uncomfortable to discuss. It is important to listen to each other. For some of us, our sexual behavior is the most serious risk to staying in recovery. For others, our sexual behavior gets us into dangerous situations that are triggers to use or drink. A few of us may have little concern about how our sexual behavior contributes to relapse. This group is an opportunity for everyone to learn about the important connection between recovery and sexual health.

LESSON INTRODUCTION

Ask another group member to volunteer to read aloud.
   The purpose of today's sexual behavior relapse prevention group is to learn about a very necessary skill for recovery. We are going to focus on sexual boundaries. We will talk about basic components of sexual boundaries with a specific focus on addressing sexual boundaries while in drug and alcohol treatment. We believe that addicts in recovery will increase their likelihood of staying sober when they develop and practice sexual boundaries that enhance and support recovery.

We will define the concepts of boundaries and sexual boundaries. We will discuss the purpose of sexual boundaries in recovery and in residential treatment. We will learn about a series of types of sexual boundaries. We will see that different sexual boundary issues have different consequences and will need to be responded to in a variety of ways. We will do several role-play and experiential exercises to rehearse and understand sexual boundaries in recovery. You will take with you "The Sexual Boundaries in Recovery Inventory" to help you determine if you have a sexual boundary issue to evaluate. This tool will assist you in addressing the sexual boundary issue.

LECTURE

Leader: Today we are going to focus on a very important topic for recovery. We are going to focus on learning about boundaries and, more specifically, sexual boundaries in recovery. We know that when people are able to set limits, to protect their bodies, to put themselves first, to say "no," to say "yes," it is essential for self-esteem, self-worth, and a general sense of feeling good about oneself.

We hope today's lesson is an opportunity to talk about and practice sexual boundary setting skills as part of reducing everyone's risk for relapse. We also want to reduce the number of people who do not successfully complete drug and alcohol treatment as a result of crossing dangerous or inappropriate sexual boundaries. In drug and alcohol treatment, some sexual boundary crossings are very harmful to the well-being and safety of all the clients, staff, and volunteers. If a sexual boundary crossing makes things dangerous, then the safety of the treatment program and its participants is first and foremost. Sometimes this means a client may be asked to leave the treatment program for the safety and well-being of everyone else at the program. This is the most severe consequence a sexual boundary violation within a drug treatment program. Our goal is to significantly decrease the likelihood of men and women in treatment who may be required to face this consequence. This lesson will provide you with information and skills about sexual boundaries. This lesson will empower you to be better prepared for setting limits and boundaries with your own sexual behavior and that of others. These boundaries will support recovery and sustain your ability to remain in drug and alcohol treatment. Healthy sexual boundaries are essential for maintaining a lifelong process for sexual health in recovery.

Let's start by talking together about the subject of boundaries. What words or phrases come to mind when you hear the word "boundaries"?

Lead a brief discussion about participants' statements. (Participants may mention topics that reflect rules, laws, basic principles from a particular religion or belief system, borders between states and countries, and being good.)

Leader: What comes to mind when you hear the phrase "sexual boundaries"?

Lead a brief discussion about participants' statements. (Group members who have attended many of the sexual health in recovery lessons may begin to review concepts from previous lessons such as sexual decisions in recovery, nonconsensual sex, and out-of-control sexual behavior. Others may emphasize boundaries just before or during sex, such as whether to have intercourse, what a person does not like to do or receive for sexual pleasure, saying "no" to sex, respecting saying "no.")

Leader: Last, what comes to mind when you think about the phrase "sexual boundaries in drug and alcohol treatment?"

Lead a brief discussion about sexual boundaries that take into consideration the risk for drinking or using drugs as a result of engaging in a certain sexual experience or not engaging in a specific sexual experience. Depending on the setting of the drug treatment program members will focus on boundaries related to group living (such as in a hospital or residential treatment setting) or boundaries related to sharing an outpatient treatment program, treatment group session, or social service recovery program. The most frequent boundaries mentioned will most likely revolve around attractions between people in a treatment program and concerns about sexual or romantic contact between patients, residents, or clients currently in the same treatment program.

Leader: As you can see, there is a lot to cover when it comes to sexual boundaries. Are there any particular associations or feelings, either positive or negative, that you have with the phrase "sexual boundaries in drug and alcohol treatment"?

Lead a discussion about common tensions surrounding sexual boundaries within a drug treatment program. Some comments may reflect the relief clients feel about having a sexual health in recovery program. Clients who have attended previous drug treatment may tell stories about how sexual concerns were restricted or unwelcome by the staff and/or other clients. Others may complain that too much emphasis is put on abstaining from relationships in the first year of recovery if a woman or man is single. Participants may have stories about previous secret or hidden relationships either in 12-step programs or within a treatment program. Some gay or lesbian clients may focus on boundaries limiting disclosure of sexual orientation. They may have fears about discussing their relationships, marriages, dating, or sexual lives within the treatment program.

Leader: I really appreciate how involved you are in wanting to offer your thoughts and feelings. When we talk about boundaries, we are talking about a particularly important subject for addicts in recovery. The very nature of addiction and maintaining an active addiction results in a multitude of failed sexual health boundaries. Why are sexual boundaries important to people in recovery? Does anyone have any ideas or thoughts about this?

Lead a brief discussion about participants' statements. Listen for participants discussing previous relapse or treatment failures that were directly linked with sex. The phrase "sex took me out the last time" may be a common experience among the group. Members may say they are in this treatment program specifically because they wanted to attend a program where sex was a welcomed topic to explore related to recovery. Others may talk about the likelihood of failing treatment if they do not really address their sex/drug-linked addiction.

EXPERIENTIAL LEARNING

Leader: *Handout "Unhealthy Boundaries" to group.* We have been using the word "boundary." How do we define "boundary"? In the handout "Unhealthy Boundaries," a boundary is defined as the personal space that you keep between yourself and others. Let's do a few exercises that give us a here and now experience with our personal space.

Create a space in the room where everyone can line up in two lines, facing each other, approximately 15 feet apart. If not enough space is available, then take participants to another location where this exercise can be conducted.

Leader: OK, let's number off by twos.

Have each group member say "one" or "two."

Leader: OK, the number ones go to the left side of the room and form a line and the number twos go to the right side and form a line.

Have participants form two lines facing each other with at least 15 feet between the two lines. If there is not an even number of participants, have two people do the exercise together with their match on the other side of the room.

Leader: Each of you choose the person directly opposite you in line to do this exercise with. Here are the directions, but do not begin the exercise until I tell you to begin. When I tell you to begin, I want you to take one step toward each other, then stop and wait for my direction. I will have you stop, look your partner in the eyes, and notice if you have any awareness of feeling uncomfortable in your personal space. (If two people are paired they each can do the exercise by stepping toward the same person.)

After you notice this, I will ask you to step forward again, look your partner in the eyes, notice your personal space, and then take another step forward. We will keep doing the exercise, moving closer to the person in the line across from you. As soon as you feel your personal space is being intruded upon, that you do not want to step any closer or have the other person step closer, put your hand out in front of you in the universal symbol for "stop." At that point both you and the person across from you will stop moving toward each other. (In the pair grouping, all three must stop as soon as one person puts his or her hand up.)

We will keep doing the exercise until there are no more dyads who can move closer to each other. Remember, the dyad stops moving closer to each other as soon as any one of the two members puts up the universal signal for stop. You must stop moving forward, whether you feel comfortable or not, if moving forward requires you to touch your partner. This exercise is a no touch exercise. Any questions?

If there are no questions, begin the exercise, making sure everyone stops after one step forward and responds to your directions. This is part of modeling good boundaries. Make sure everyone is following the directions. Do not let anyone move ahead of the directions. Continue exercise until everyone is finished. Have a discussion of what people noticed about their personal space. What body, visual, or thought cues did they use to gauge their personal space? Discuss the importance of honoring when someone says "stop," even though you may have still been comfortable to keep going.

Leader: OK, let's do this again, only this time, when the first person in the dyad puts up the universal sign for stop, only the person putting up the stop sign will no longer move forward. The other person in the dyad will continue moving forward, following my directions, until he or she wants to stop. (If there is a triad, the members keep moving forward until all three have decided to stop.) Then that person will put up the stop sign. You must stop moving forward, whether you feel comfortable or not, if moving forward requires you to touch your partner. This exercise is a no touch exercise. Any questions?

Repeat exercise, same as before, until all participants have stop sign up or can no longer move because of the no touch rule.

Leader: What does it feel like to have someone keep moving toward you even though you wanted him or her to stop? What does it feel like to have someone say stop and for you to keep moving?

Have a discussion from both points of view.

Leader: OK, let's do this exercise one more time but with a bit of a twist. I want you imagine that the person you are walking toward is someone to whom you feel an attraction. Don't worry if the gender of the person you are moving toward is not the gender you are oriented to sexually. This is a pretend exercise. You will each follow the same directions, except neither of you will stop based on your personal space. I am handing out sheets of paper with numbers on them. Each person in line one will get a number.

Give each person in line a number. Assign numbers randomly. Several of the dyads may have the same number. Dyads will only stop moving when you call out their number. The point of this exercise is for participants to feel the randomness and unexpectedness of when they will need to stop. Let some of the dyads go well past the previously established comfort zones.

Leader: When I say your number out loud, you will put up the stop sign and no longer mover toward your partner. Your partner will stop as well. We will complete the exercise until everyone has stopped. No one will be allowed to touch each other. I will make sure you all stop before you must touch. Any questions?

Complete third part of exercise.

Leader: What does it feel like to not be in control of when you stopped, but to have it controlled by your number?

Have a discussion among all participants.

Leader: Each of these three experiences is an opportunity to experience the three kinds of boundary issues we are going to talk about in this lesson. Remember these experiences for our next discussion.

There are three levels of boundary issues we are going to talk about (Gutheil & Brodsky, 2008). This means that there are different degrees of seriousness of boundaries and different levels of feelings and consequences when these different levels of boundaries are crossed. The three levels are:

1. Boundary challenges
2. Boundary crossings
3. Boundary violations

The first exercise we did was an example of a boundary challenge. In the first exercise we had someone put up the stop sign and the partner then stopped and no one moved after that. A boundary challenge is when one person is very clear about his or her boundary and clearly communicates the boundary, like putting up his or her hand with the universal stop signal. The other person is given the challenge. The person being told to stop has the challenge of either choosing to cooperate and respect and honor the request of the other person or not. This is a challenge. We have so many of these events throughout our day that we probably cannot keep track of them all.

What are some examples of boundaries you need to set among fellow clients at a drug treatment program? Put another way, when do one or more people say "stop" in one form or another and the person being told to stop has to decide whether to honor the request?

Have a discussion of day-to-day living issues if the treatment program is residential. Discuss things like sharing the bathroom, dressing, undressing, snoring, meal time, chores, loudness of voice, taking phone messages, showing up for duties, meetings, asking to borrow money, and so forth. Reinforce the idea that in order to live here and be in a recovery community together, everyone is agreeing to honor and respect other people's boundaries in various situations all day. If the program is an outpatient program, boundaries may focus less on details of sharing space 24 hours a day. Participants may focus on issues around confidentiality, disclosure about what is said in treatment to others outside of the program, judgmental responses to risk taking in group sessions, and seeing each other at 12-step programs or out in the community.

Leader: Boundary challenges are not a sign of a problem. In fact, if the only boundary situations you face all day are boundary challenges, then you are having a pretty good day. Boundary challenges are part of the normal expectations of life. The boundary challenges we discussed here are all part of the usual boundary concerns within a drug and alcohol treatment program. If we are having difficulty with boundary challenges, then the other two boundary issues will be very stressful and could be a significant factor in relapse.

Of all the boundary challenges we talked about, take a moment to think about which sexual boundary challenge is especially important to you. I will give you a moment to think about this. OK, would anyone like to share what sexual boundary challenge they thought was especially important to them?

Have a brief discussion. Give several people a chance to share what they came up with.

Leader: The most important thing to notice is that a day-to-day sexual boundary challenge that may be really important to you may not be the same importance for someone else. Being a resident, patient, or client in drug treatment requires us to communicate the sexual boundary challenges that are important to each of us. We believe that failing to negotiate these daily sexual challenges can make participating in treatment very stressful.

TOPIC SKILL PRACTICE

Leader: One way to improve our skills at negotiating sexual boundary challenges is to practice in front of a group. I want to give some of you an opportunity to role-play a sexual boundary challenge and get feedback from the class about your approach. We can do either a role-play that you think will show the group some good skills for handling a sexual boundary challenge or you can volunteer because you want to get better at handling a particular situation more effectively. Does anyone have a situation they would like to role-play? You can choose to be whichever person in the role-play you want to be. I will ask for a volunteer from the class to be the other person in the role-play.

> *Choose a volunteer, have him explain the situation clearly, have him explain if this is a demonstration of a skill he feels good about or whether he wants help. Have him choose one goal for the role-play, such as "I want to show how I handle someone walking in on me when I am using the bathroom" or "I want to stop someone from borrowing my clothes to go on a date without asking me." Have him choose the role he wants to play and have a volunteer do the other part. Have each role-play last no longer than 3–4 minutes. Discuss reactions, thoughts, and focus on what either person did well. Focus on the strengths, good choices, or useful responses. Highlight the importance of handling these situations early before they reach a more serious level.*
>
> *Look for several key components of role-play and process the key boundary setting skills after the role-play. Key components are:*
>
> ■ *How did the person phrase the boundary challenge? Did he or she state an understandable brief statement describing the boundary challenge. "I don't like you telling me what Sam said at the AA meeting last night," "I would prefer shaking hands with you rather than hug when we meet," or "Will you make sure to knock on the bedroom door before entering if the door is closed."*
> ■ *Discuss if the boundary is a physical space boundary or an emotional space boundary. Utilize the boundary exercise to describe a physical space boundary. How close we want people to be is a physical space boundary. An emotional space boundary is how you felt when you were having eye contact while standing and moving in the line. Eye contact is a very common emotional space boundary.*
> ■ *Lastly, discuss how the receiver of the boundary challenge responded. Did the person listen, get defensive, or try to explain the behavior? Focus on how boundary challenges require respect from both people involved in the interaction.*
>
> *Review these three components after discussing the role-play.*
>
> 1. *Is it an understandable clear brief statement?*
> 2. *Is it an emotional or physical boundary challenge?*
> 3. *Was the boundary challenge respectfully stated and listened to?*

Leader: The second level of boundary issues are boundary crossings.

A boundary crossing is when your own emotional limits or personal space boundary is crossed by another person. Remember a boundary crossing is when the limits in the relationship are adjusted or altered. This can lead to confusion and uncertainty. Someone may be physically closer, emotionally closer, or mentally closer than you want him or her to be. The previously established boundary has been altered. When a boundary has been altered without our consent, we usually have feelings and reactions. Sometimes we feel confused or uncertain about what to do, and a lack of clarity, feelings of doubt, or tension may occur.

Remember what you felt in the exercise when you wanted your partner to stop because your personal space was being intruded upon, but your partner was able to continue forward. Boundary crossings are almost always a situation where one person's boundary is very different from another's boundary. A boundary crossing is an important relationship moment where people need to stop and talk and renegotiate the boundary between them. The solution to this difference may be harmful if one of the people tries to overpower the other person, ignore his or her boundary, or try to get him or her to alter his or her boundary by coercion, manipulation, deception, or lies. These are very common behaviors that addicts use to maintain their addictions. These are also common sexual boundary crossings men and women do in order to maintain their addictions. Let's think aloud with each other of examples of common sexual boundary crossings of alcoholic or drug-addicted men and women.

Have a discussion that involves examples of boundary crossings, in which someone has set a sexual boundary and the other person attempts to get the person to change his or her boundary. Examples might include:

- *Trying to get someone to have sex without the use of condoms for sexually transmitted infection (STI) protection or to prevent an unwanted pregnancy.*
- *Having sex with someone else's boyfriend or girlfriend and convincing him or her to keep it a secret.*
- *Making offensive sexual comments.*
- *Continuously inserting sexualized talk and humor into conversations.*
- *Telling explicit sexual stories or adventures.*
- *Asking intrusive sexual questions.*
- *The general theme is sexual situations where the addict is invested in getting someone to cross a boundary that he or she really does not want to cross.*

Leader: OK, now what would be some examples of physical sexual boundary crossing that may happen at this treatment center? The previous boundary crossings were emotional. Now let's focus on physical sexual boundary crossings that can happen between clients or between clients and staff at this treatment center. The first physical boundary to consider is touch. Remember that we have certain boundaries about touch here. What are ways that people can cross these touch boundaries?

Have a similar discussion. Keep the distinction between a boundary crossing and violation. Violations are much more severe and always cause harm. A boundary crossing causes tension, anxiety, but at least one person in the situation has control over the situation. Remind them that in the exercise each person had a choice to make about when to stop moving based on his or her own personal space. Emphasize situations where sexual talk, flirting, seductive contact, and so forth still allows each person a choice on how to respond.

Leader: Of all the boundary crossings we talked about, take a moment to think about which sexual boundary crossing is especially important to you. Think about which sexual boundary crossing would have a serious emotional consequence for you if you continue to allow the boundary to be crossed. Think about which sexual boundary crossing would be so emotionally upsetting that your mind may begin to have thoughts about using. Perhaps the sexual boundary crossing is a common boundary crossing that happened all the time when you were drinking or getting high. Knowing what one key sexual boundary crossing may increase your risk for relapse is an excellent tool for sexual health in recovery. I will give you a moment to think about this. OK, would anyone like to share what sexual boundary crossing they thought was especially important to them?

Have a brief discussion and give several people a chance to share what they came up with.

Leader: The most important thing to notice is that a sexual boundary crossing that may be really important to you may not be the same importance for someone else. A drug treatment center situation requires us to communicate sexual boundary crossings. This is a key for sexual health in recovery to begin with the onset of treatment. A treatment center that can respectfully negotiate sexual boundary crossings between any and every person, whether between clients, between client and counselor, or any other combination is laying the foundation for a sex-positive treatment environment. When sexual boundary crossings are not effectively addressed, even more serious and perhaps unsafe sexual situations may emerge. We believe that clients and staff failing to respond effectively to sexual boundary crossings can lead to sexual violations.

I want give some of you an opportunity to role-play a sexual boundary crossing and get feedback from the class about your approach. We can do either a role-play that you think will show the group some good skills for handling a sexual boundary crossing or you can volunteer because you want to get better at handling a particular situation more effectively. Does anyone have a situation they would like to role-play? You can choose to be whichever person in the role-play you want to be. I will ask for a volunteer from the class to be the other person in the role-play.

Repeat as with previous role-play.

- *How did the person phrase the boundary crossing? Did he or she state an understandable brief statement describing the boundary crossing? "Please don't squeeze my bottom when you hug me at meetings," "Please close the bathroom door when you are showering," "I am uncomfortable with you telling me about what online sex sites you like to use," or "Please do not ask me to keep a secret about having sex with the staff member who no longer works here."*
- *Discuss if the boundary is a physical space boundary crossing or an emotional space boundary crossing. Utilize the boundary exercise to describe a physical space boundary. How close we want people to be is a physical space boundary. An emotional space boundary is how you felt when the person kept moving and you had put up the signal to stop or you kept moving toward a person who had asked you to stop coming closer.*
- *Last, discuss how both people listened and made an honest attempt to negotiate the boundary. Did both people listen, get defensive, or try to maintain their boundary crossing behavior? Did the discussion lead to a return to a better boundary? Focus on how boundary crossing discussion requires an expression of feelings and expression of respect between both people involved in the interaction.*

Review these three components after discussing the role-play.

1. *Is it an understandable clear brief statement?*
2. *Is it an emotional or physical boundary challenge*
3. *Was the boundary crossing respectfully negotiated?*

Leader: Boundary violations are the most severe and always result in harm. Boundary violations cause harm and pain because the control of one's boundaries was relinquished to someone else. A person will commit a boundary violation only if he or she is interested in exerting a significant amount of power over another person and needs to engage in harm by doing one of two things:

1. Physical or sexual boundary intrusion
2. Emotional boundary intrusion

Let's talk for a bit about each one of these.

Sexual intrusions are violations that breach a physical or emotional boundary. A physical boundary is defined by our skin, body, and self. I decide how I am touched, who touches me, and where I am touched. An emotional boundary is defined by our age, relationship with those around us, our personal requirements for safety, and how we want to be treated. In other words, an emotional boundary is about choosing how I want people to treat me. I can set limits on what people say to me. I can determine what kind of personal feedback and comments I will accept from others. Even if I let someone do something once that I did not like, I can change my mind and not let him or her do it again. I can set a new standard or boundary for myself after thinking about a previous situation. I can determine how much personal information I will reveal to others.

Write the words physical or sexual boundary violation followed by emotional boundary violation on the board. Ask group for examples of each. Add examples of each as participants offer them.

Leader: What are some examples that come to mind of a physical or sexual boundary intrusion?

Request examples from group. Examples might include the following:

- *Incest,*
- *Sexual abuse,*
- *Rape,*
- *Inappropriate touching,*
- *Infecting someone who does not want to become infected with HIV or STIs,*
- *Having sex with another person in the treatment program,*

- *Having sex with a newcomer at AA/NA,*
- *Voyeurism,*
- *Recording someone having sex without his or her consent,*
- *Showing videos of someone having sex without his or her consent,*
- *Sending nude or sexual pictures of someone on the Internet without his or her consent,*
- *Giving someone drugs to get him or her high in order to have sex with him or her,*
- *Sex with a minor, and*
- *Showing sexual images or sex videos to minors and children.*

Leader: What are some examples that come to mind of emotional boundary intrusions?

Request examples from group. Examples might include the following:

- *Inappropriate personal questions to someone you do not know very well,*
- *Disclosing aspects of your sexual life indiscriminately in groups for many people to overhear, and*
- *Disclosing personal or confidential information to other people.*

Leader: OK, now what would be some examples of sexual boundary violations that may happen at this treatment center? Remember that we have certain boundaries about touch here. What are ways that people can violate these touch boundaries?

Have a similar discussion. Keep the distinction between a boundary crossing and violation. Violations are much more severe and always cause harm. Remind them that in the last of the three boundary experiential exercises, neither of the people in the dyad had a choice of when they got to stop. Their internal feelings of personal space being violated did not determine when each person stopped moving toward each other. This is the most important distinction between a sexual boundary crossing and a violation. In a violation, there is at least one or more people who have not given consent but must suffer a painful consequence as a result. It is the survivor of the violation who bears the brunt of the emotional shock.

Leader: Of all the boundary violations we talked about, take a moment to think about which sexual boundary violation is especially important to you. I will give you a moment to think about this. Think about which sexual boundary violations would cause serious harm.

Think about which sexual boundary violation would be so emotionally or physically harmful that your mind may immediately want to stop thinking about this violation and think about using or drinking. Perhaps the sexual boundary violation happened only in situations involving sex and drugs. Knowing one key sexual boundary violation that only is connected with sex and drugs combined can be an important sexual health in recovery tool. It can be very comforting to remind yourself that as long as you stay clean and sober you do not have much worry about this sexual violation happening again.

Pause, let group contemplate this moment before returning to discussion.

Leader: OK, would anyone like to share what sexual violation crossing they thought was especially important to them?

Have a brief discussion, and give several people a chance to share what they came up with

Leader: A sexual boundary violation can be accidental or can be done out of kindness, and it can be a result of being thoughtless, intentional, or malicious. We believe that failing to effectively respond to sexual boundary violations can lead to relapse. Sexual boundary violations create an unsafe treatment environment and harm clients, staff, and the recovery process. Sexual boundary violations interfere with the ability to receive effective and safe drug and alcohol treatment, and such violations contribute significantly to treatment failure or relapse and can lead to possible death from overdose, violence, and crime.

Before we do a few role-plays, let's talk about sexual boundary distance violations. A distance violation is when closeness and understanding in a relationship is cut off when you have a realistic expectation or even right to expect closeness. An abrupt or sudden extreme distance in a relationship can be harmful. A person might see his or her close friend in treatment crying and just walk by and act like nothing is happening. You might overhear someone planning to go out and use and say nothing to the person. You may know someone is planning to do something dangerous to harm him or herself—perhaps he or she confided in you that he or she is thinking of attempting suicide—and you do nothing with the information and go about your day. What are some other examples that may come to mind that describe sexual boundary violations of distance?

Write them on the board.

Leader: We are not going to role-play sexual boundary violations. We are going to role-play how to reach out for help in response to a sexual boundary violation. Getting help from a trusted person is an essential response following a boundary violation. Too often someone will want to address the person who has violated his or her boundary without seeking emotional support and guidance first. The sexual health in recovery skill we want to practice in these role-plays is how to seek support following a boundary violation. This is not a moment to process an actual boundary violation in your life. This is a role-play to practice three skills. If you cannot do the role play without using the role-play to process a sexual violation in your life, then I ask that you pass on this invitation and let another group member do the exercise for us.

The role-play can either show the group some good skills for approaching someone for support following a sexual boundary violation or it can demonstrate how to begin discussing the actual sexual boundary violation with your chosen helper. Does anyone have a situation they would like to role-play? You can choose to be whichever person in the role-play you want to be. I will ask for a volunteer from the class to be the other person in the role-play.

> *Repeat as with previous role-play.*
>
> *How did the person phrase the boundary violation? Did he or she state an understandable brief statement describing the boundary violation? "My roommate was masturbating in bed last night and asked if I wanted to watch," "My counselor asked me out on a date," "Another person (name) in the treatment program is having sex with my sponsor and threatened to tell my husband about my secret abortion I had 13 years ago if I told anyone," "I just found out that the man I had sex with last week is HIV-positive and he lied to me when I asked him," or "My daughter told me that my last boyfriend who was also my dealer was forcing her to give him oral sex."*
>
> *Discuss how the person is doing and what he or she needs from the helper at this very moment. Last, discuss how both people listened and did not react immediately to the disclosure. The focus was on the immediate emotional, physical, and safety needs of the person who was violated. Focus on what boundaries the person who was violated needs from the helper*
>
> *Review these three components after discussing the role-play.*

1. *Is it an understandable clear brief statement?*
2. *Focus on what the person needs from the helper.*
3. *Are you safe? Are you hurt? How are you feeling?*

Leader: I am now handing out a simple worksheet you can use to improve your abilities in setting sexual boundaries. "The Sexual Boundaries in Recovery Inventory" is a tool to help you determine if you have a sexual boundary issue to address as well as a simple guide to assist you in addressing the boundary issue. You can refer to this list if you notice yourself feeling angry, upset, irritated, embarrassed, ashamed, resentful, anxious, or other uncomfortable feelings. Check in with yourself to see if these feelings have anything to do a sexual boundary issue. Identifying a sexual boundary issue is a very important skill. Many times we are unaware that a sexual boundary has been challenged or crossed. We have proposed that if you do not address these sexual boundary challenges and sexual boundary crossings, you may be placing yourself at increased risk for relapse related to a sexual violation.

Hand out "The Sexual Boundaries in Recovery Inventory" (Lesson 11 appendix, B). Review the directions for the sheet and discuss any questions people may have about using it.

CLOSING

Leader: Now let's take a moment to bring the workshop to a close. Let's take a moment to again quiet ourselves, take a deep breath to quiet our minds, our hearts, and our spirits. In this quiet place, remind yourself how valuable it is to take the time to be honest, vulnerable, and committed to recovery. As you leave the group today, remind yourself that a satisfying sexual life is a vital and important part of recovery. The self-reflection and tools you learned today may become an important part of maintaining your recovery.

REFERENCES

Covington, S. (2000). *Awakening your sexuality: A guide for recovering women.* Center City, MN: Hazelden.

Gutheil, T., & Brodsky, A. (2008). *Preventing boundary violations in clinical practice.* New York: Guilford Press.

Katherine, A. (1993). *Boundaries: Where you end and I begin.* New York: Simon and Schuster.

Nelson, P. (1993). *There's a hole in my sidewalk: The romance of self-discovery.* Hillsboro, OR: Beyond Words Publishing.

Peter, V., & Dowd, T. (2000). *Boundaries: A guide for teens.* Boys Town, NE: The Boys Town Press.

Wagner, R. (Director). (2006). *Boundaries: Stop getting abused and learn healthy boundaries* [VHS and DVD]. United States: Asktheinternetthrapist.com.

Wertheimer, A. (2003). *Consent to sexual relations.* Cambridge, UK: Cambridge University Press.

LESSON 11 APPENDIX

A. Unhealthy Boundaries

A boundary is the personal space that you keep between yourself and others. Boundaries let everyone know your areas of privacy.

Sexual and Physical Boundaries Protect Our Bodies
- Who can touch you?
- How can they touch you?
- Where can another person touch you?

Emotional and Spiritual Boundaries Protect Private Thoughts and Emotions
- What feelings do I want to share with this person?
- What feelings am I not ready to share?
- Who are the people I trust with my deepest feelings?

Characteristics of rigid boundaries: These can lead to isolation and loneliness, keeping people very distant, and not letting anyone get close.

1. Whenever possible avoid talking about personal feelings.
2. Whenever possible avoid talking about personal needs.
3. Whenever possible avoid talking about deep emotions and feelings with recovery support network.
4. Difficulty keeping friends
5. Difficulty choosing friends
6. Avoid close relationships

Characteristics of too loose or weak boundaries: These can lead to hurt and pain.

1. Displaying inappropriate affection.
2. Whenever possible avoid saying "no."
3. Whenever possible avoid disagreeing.
4. Whenever possible go along with what others say or want.
5. Say or do sexually suggestive things in front of others.
6. Share too much personal information about yourself.
7. Share personal information about yourself before you are ready.
8. Being tricked into being used or abused.

9. Whenever possible avoid conflict.
10. Having many sexual experiences.
11. Continuing with a sexual experience even though you don't want to.
12. Taking responsibility for others' feelings.

The following are behavioral examples of people violating your boundaries:

1. Interrupting your conversations.
2. Taking your possessions.
3. Teasing that hurts you.
4. Asking personal questions that are inappropriate.
5. Gossiping about you.
6. Always hanging around you and invading your private space.
7. Saying offensive or vulgar things.
8. Doing offensive or vulgar things.
9. Always trying to sit or stand too close to you.
10. Forcing you to do something sexual.
11. Physically abusing you.
12. Sexually abusing you.
13. Inappropriate language and touch.

Some content adapted from Peter and Dowd (2000).

B. The Sexual Boundaries in Recovery Inventory

Take a few minutes to reflect on your day. Did you experience any sexual boundary issues today? The checklist offers a few examples of sexual boundary challenges, sexual boundary crossings, and sexual boundary violations. If you experienced a boundary challenge, crossing, or violation, check your level of concern in response to this boundary issue.

Remember the sequence for resolving any sexual boundary issue is:

1. The sexual boundary issue is identified and described clearly.
2. Talk about the boundary issue with the person who was involved in the boundary challenge or crossing. Talk with a trusted helper after a boundary violation.
3. The boundary challenger, or crosser, listens and negotiates a resolution. The helper asks if your are safe, if you are hurt, and how you are feeling.

Sexual Boundary Challenges	Very concerned	Somewhat concerned	No concern

Sharing the bathroom.

Interrupts when you are talking.

Talks about him or herself without asking how your are doing.

Makes sexual jokes in response to sex/drug-linked relapse concerns.

_____

_____

Sexual Boundary Crossings	Very concerned	Somewhat concerned	No concern

Offensive sexual comments.

Being constantly sexualized.

Sexual stories or exploits.

Intrusive sexual questions.

Gossiping about client's sex life.

_____

_____

Sexual Boundary Violations	Very concerned	Somewhat concerned	No concern
Sex with another client.			
Sex with a newcomer to AA/NA.			
Sponsor wanting to have sex.			
Counselor asked me for a date.			
Masturbated with someone in the treatment program.			
Sex that could lead to contracting HIV or another STI.			

_____

_____

Definitions

Sexual boundary challenges: One person is very clear about his or her boundary and clearly communicates the boundary or request. The other person is given the challenge. The person listening to the request has the challenge of choosing to cooperate, respect, and honor the request. This is sexual boundary challenge.

Sexual boundary crossings: Your own sexual limits, boundaries, or personal sexual space are crossed by another person. He or she is physically closer, emotionally closer, or mentally closer than you want him or her to be. The previously established sexual boundary has been altered. When a sexual boundary has been altered without our consent, we usually have feelings and reactions.

Sexual boundary violations: These are the most severe sexual violations, and they always result in harm. Harm and pain results from the loss of control of one's boundaries. Violations of sexual intrusion can happen by breaching a physical or emotional boundary. A physical boundary is defined by our skin, body, and self. I decide how I am touched, who touches me, and where I am touched. An emotional boundary is defined our age, role, relationship with those around us, our personal requirements for safety, and how we want to be treated.

Remember: "Boundaries bring order to our lives. As we learn to strengthen our boundaries, we gain a clearer sense of ourselves and our relationship to others. Boundaries empower us to determine how we'll be treated by others. With good boundaries, we can have the wonderful assurance that comes from knowing we can and will protect ourselves from the ignorance, meanness, and thoughtlessness of others" (Katherine, 1993, p. 17).

12

Relationship with My Body

CORE CONCEPT

A frequent motivator for the use of drugs and alcohol is to reduce, eliminate, or alter our feelings and thoughts about our body in order to experience sexual pleasure or functioning. Chemically dependent women and men rely on drugs and alcohol to alter or influence their body image to feel sexual or attractive or to express their sexual desires. Men and women with high sex/drug-linked addiction may be unprepared to address their link between body image and their drug and alcohol abuse. Sexual health in drug and alcohol treatment includes facing body image conflicts and shame to maintain abstinence. The first section of this module provides a group experience to discuss body shame as a collective experience that men and women share to some degree. The remainder of the class will be conducted in separate women's and men's groups. The "Body Self-Talk in Recovery" assessment reinforces self-awareness of self-talk body statements directly linked with personal history of drug and alcohol abuse.

BELIEF STATEMENT

Sexual health in recovery is the ability to maintain a positive body image.

OBJECTIVES

Participants will

- Discuss common body image attitudes among men and women.
- Discuss common uses of drugs and alcohol to alter body image attitudes.
- Learn about negative and positive self-statements about one's body.
- Learn to use the "Body Self-Talk in Recovery" assessment tool.

CHANGE GOALS

- Link drug use history with body image and body attitude conflicts,
- Increase awareness of negative and positive self-talk about one's body.
- Utilize "Body Self-Talk in Recovery" to assess risk for relapse as it pertains to body image.

REQUIRED READING FOR GROUP LEADER

- *Body Image: Understanding Body Dissatisfaction in Men, Women and Children* by Sarah Grogan (2008) is a comprehensive overview of current theory, research, and treatment approaches for children and adults dissatisfied with their bodies. Grogan provides clear definitions of terms and cites a wide breadth of research and current clinical understanding of addressing body image concerns. She also addresses both male and female body image dissatisfaction. It is essential for the sexual health in recovery group leader to be familiar with gender-influenced similarities and differences of body image. This book will provide group leaders with significant background material to lead either the male or female breakout groups in this lesson.
- In our experience at Stepping Stone, where this curriculum was first piloted, the body image lesson was consistently rated as a top favorite. Shame about body image may be much more closely linked among the men and women in recovery and therefore a significant relapse prevention intervention. It only makes sense that the very vessel in which we experience sexual feelings, contact, and

pleasure is central to sex itself. If one is feeling dissatisfied with the original contact point for sex, our body, then the remainder of negotiation for sexual health will be fraught with tension. Being prepared for the deep meaning of body image conflicts among men and women in recovery is a primary leadership skill for this lesson.

- *Sex Matters for Women: A Complete Guide to Taking Care of Your Sexual Self* includes a chapter on body image (Foley, Kope, & Sugrue, 2002). I expanded on the authors' concept of utilizing the couples work of John Gottman (Gottman & Silver, 1999; Gottman, Gottman & DeClaire, 2006) as a relationship strategy for addressing punitive negative body self-talk to create the "Body Self-Talk in Recovery" worksheet.

- *The Seven Principles for Making Marriage Work* (Gottman & Silver, 1999) outlines four kinds of negative interactions between couples that, when they persist, are "lethal" to a relationship (Gottman & Silver, 1999, p. 27). I have adapted these negative interactions as they pertain to our own opinions about our bodies. Lethal persistent body image thoughts, perceptions, and behaviors contradict the basic elements of recovery. This conflict may lead to increased risk for relapse, especially when entering or reentering an active sexual life in recovery. Leaders who become familiar with the language Gottman and Silver have named "The Four Horseman of the Apocalypse" (1999, p. 27)—criticism, contempt, defensiveness, and stonewalling—will recognize the integration of these within the basic structure of the lesson as well as the "Body Self-Talk in Recovery" worksheet. In this lesson I utilized Gottman's remedy of transforming a criticism into a complaint, combined with the additional remedy of thinking positively about the body. Gottman's research is integral to understanding this lesson.

REQUIRED MATERIALS FOR THE LESSON

- An mp3 player and music selection
- Blackboard, white board, or flip chart
- Posters with body parts written on them (see experiential learning exercise)
- 3 × 5 cards (four for each participant)

- Basket or container to collect cards
- "Body Self-Talk in Recovery" worksheet (one copy for each participant) (Lesson 12 appendix)

OPENING

Opening Music: *Have quiet music playing as participants enter the room and ready themselves (optional).*

Leader: As we sit quietly and focus on being here, let us clear our minds of where we have been and focus on being in this moment.

Opening Poem/Reading:

Sex contains all, bodies,
souls, Meanings, proofs, purities, delicacies, results, promulgations,
Songs, commands, health, pride, the maternal mystery, the seminal milk,
All hopes, benefactions, bestowals, all the passions, loves, beauties,
delights of the earth,
All the governments, judges, gods, follow'd persons of the earth,
These are contained in sex as parts of itself and justifications of itself.
Without shame the man I like knows and avows
the deliciousness of his sex,
Without shame the woman I like knows and avows hers . . .

—Walt Whitman, "A Woman Waits for Me,"
Leaves of Grass

GROUP INTRODUCTION

Have group member volunteer to read aloud.

Welcome to the sexual health in recovery group. We are here to talk about sex and how our sexual lives affect recovery from drug and alcohol addiction. Some people in recovery risk a relapse because of their sexual behavior at the treatment center or away from the treatment program. This is a place to talk about sexual behavior and sexual health so we can be abstinent from drugs and alcohol. It is also a place to learn about sexual behavior and situations that put men and women in recovery at risk for not completing this treatment program.

Sexual health in recovery is a time to talk about human sexuality and sexual health in a respectful and informed manner. We encourage everyone to be as honest and open as you can be. You are not required to reveal anything about your current or past sexual behavior that would be uncomfortable to discuss. It is important to listen to each other. For some of us, our sexual behavior is the most serious risk to staying in recovery. For others, our sexual behavior gets us into dangerous situations that are triggers to use or drink. A few of us may have little concern about how our sexual behavior contributes to relapse. This group is an opportunity for everyone to learn about the important connection between recovery and sexual health.

LESSON INTRODUCTION

Ask another group member to volunteer to read aloud.

The purpose of today's sexual behavior relapse prevention group is to learn about how early recovery is an important time to attend to your personal relationship with your body. We will discuss how a negative relationship with our bodies may have significantly motivated our abuse and eventual addiction to drugs and alcohol. Sexual health in recovery believes women and men in recovery will increase their likelihood of staying sober when they maintain a positive body image.

Together we will explore the connection between body image and drug and alcohol use. We will create a list of desirable and undesirable features of many body parts. We will refine these lists to identify the link between living with undesirable body features and drug and alcohol addiction. We will then separate into separate men's and women's groups. Each group will learn about how our body self-talk can have profound effects on our sexual health in recovery. We will learn that one negative body thought will need five positive thoughts as a counterbalance. Not enough positive self-talk statements will lead to an unsatisfactory and unfulfilling relationship with your body. We will practice using the "Body Self-Talk in Recovery" worksheet to identify destructive body self-talk and utilize proven relationship skills to minimize the harm from negative body self-talk.

LECTURE

Leader: Talk about a love/hate relationship! Is there any more complicated relationship we have had our entire lives than the relationship we have with our bodies? The body is a home, yet almost every element in society tries to tell us whether it is attractive, acceptable, and living up to an impossible standard. We are going to spend time together looking at how our relationship with our body is linked with our use of drugs and alcohol. For men and women in recovery it is vital to understand their motivation for using specific drugs to alter their relationship with their bodies. The drug-induced high may have allowed them to have sex, to enjoy sex, to alleviate shame before, during, or after sex, to prolong sexual activity, to feel attractive, to perform or receive a specific sexual act, and/or to sexually function. This workshop will focus on our own body image and how we may have attempted to change our body image by using drugs or drinking.

EXPERIENTIAL LEARNING

Leader: What do we mean by the phrase "body image"?

Take ideas from the class.

Leader: Body image is defined by Sarah Grogan as "a person's perceptions, thoughts, and feelings about his or her body" (Grogan, 2008, p. 3). Body image is a basic part of our identity and our self-concept. Researchers (Davison & McCabe, 2005) have found that women who are disappointed and unhappy with their body image tend to focus on their overall body shape, especially their hips, waist, and thighs. Men who are dissatisfied with their body image tend to focus on their height, stomach, chest, and hair loss.

Let's do our own experiment and see what everyone in this room thinks. We have pieces of paper posted around the room with the names of a body part or function.

Place posters around the room. Each one should list a particular body part most associated with body shame in women and in men: for women, it is their body shape, hips, waist, and thighs. For men it is height, stomach, chest, and hair loss. Under each body part or function are two columns, one titled "attractive" and the other "unattractive."

Leader: Under each body part or function are two columns. One is titled "attractive," and the other is "unattractive." We want you to move about the room and write under each body part or function a feature of that body part or function that is commonly thought of as attractive or a feature that is commonly considered unattractive. Don't worry if it may be more specific to men or women. We are not concerned about gender differences at this point in the workshop. We just want to spend some time discussing these very common attitudes and ideas we all carry around with us about our bodies.

Let's do an example together before we begin. Let's say the body part or function is "eyes."

Write "eyes" on the white board, with two columns underneath, one labeled "attractive" and one "unattractive."

Leader: What are some common desirable features of eyes?

Call on participants and write answers in the "attractive" column. Have answers be very brief (1–4 words). This is important, because most body image thoughts are quite brief, short, and to the point. For "eyes," people may say things like: a certain color, big, expressive, not too small, and so forth. When this is completed, move on to the "unattractive" column.

Leader: OK, what are some examples of undesirable features of eyes?

Do similar exercise.

Leader: OK, here are a couple of suggestions before we begin. Let's all move as a circle around the room, going from each word to the next without jumping ahead in line. If you do not have something to write for the word in front of you, wait until the person ahead of you moves on to the next word. If someone has written what you wanted to write, see if you can come up with something else, or just put a check mark next to the duplicate answer. We will do this until everyone has had a chance to move about the circle and answer each word. Any questions before we get started?

Answer any lingering questions before beginning.

Leader: OK, let's all stand up and make room for our circle to move about the room. Stand in a circle, and I will let you know when we are ready to begin. Make sure everyone has a pen. OK, let's begin.

Let exercise go for as long as it takes group to go around the room once. When everyone is finished, have them return to their seats.

Leader: Before we discuss what you have written, I want you all to look around the room at the various comments that everyone has written. Which items do you relate to? Which undesirable body features or body functioning do you worry about in yourself? Which specific body features or functioning are you pleased about with yourself?

I am passing around four 3 × 5 cards. On one card, I want you to write one body feature or function you find undesirable about yourself. Write only one, not more than one. On the other card, I want you to write five body features or functions you find desirable about yourself. Do not write less than five; do not write more than five. Just five. Leave the other two cards blank. After you have written your responses on two cards, place them in the basket in the center of the room. We are going to read these aloud together, but we will not identify who wrote them. If you do not want what you have written on the card read aloud, then turn in the two cards you have left blank and keep your written cards for yourself.

Have the participants complete the exercise and turn in the cards.

Leader: I will now walk around the room and have you take two cards from the basket. It doesn't matter if you get two cards with an undesirable or desirable list. It does not matter if you get one of your own cards. It does not matter if you get one or two blank cards. You will know if the description is undesirable because it has only one answer. You will know it is desirable because it has five answers. Hold your cards privately to yourself. We will get to them in just a bit.

Now, we will do the same circle exercise with the body parts written on the wall. This time, as we walk around the room with our pens, you will circle any body function or part that is associated with *you using drugs or alcohol*. Write the name of the drug or drug(s) that may be used to cope with this undesirable or desirable body part or feature. The drug may be legal, illegal, prescription or nonprescription, addictive or non-addictive. The main point is that drugs or alcohol were used to cope with your feelings or to try to change, improve, or maintain the body feature. You may have used these drugs to change how this body part functioned. Drugs may have been an attempt to tune out the punitive, hateful chatter in your mind so you could function sexually. For example, someone may have taken crystal meth to lose weight. Notice as you go around the room that some of the items will be associated with drugs and alcohol, while others may not. Remember, just circle the item, even if the item is already circled; just circle it again. The more circles, the more members of our class may have associated that body part or function with drugs and alcohol. Any questions before we begin?

Allow time for questions before doing exercise same as the previous exercise.

Leader: OK, let's begin.

Let exercise go for as long as it takes group to go around the room once. When everyone is finished, have them return to their seats.

Leader: OK, now let's look at the body image/drug-linked associations that people circled. These are body image and body relationship issues that may be associated with addiction and therefore are also related to recovery. Let's look at what people circled. What are your thoughts, reactions, or comments about what you see on our lists?

Sarah Grogan (2008) summarizes key body image issues for women and men. Women may focus more on areas of their body where fat accumulates; look for women to focus on thighs, buttocks, hips, and mid-torso. Look for associations with drugs and alcohol related to these body areas and dissatisfaction. Conversely, women may be less preoccupied with the top half of their body; see if less drug and alcohol links are made for these body areas with women.

Notice if the women or gay men are more focused on body image satisfaction than the heterosexual men and lesbian participants. Gay men strongly acculturated within the gay community may mirror body image issues more closely associated with heterosexually identified women. Lesbians may think they are expected to be less body focused yet may privately be focused on weight and fitness to a degree they do not easily discuss.

Heterosexual men tend to less preoccupied in general with body image concerns and tend to report much more positive body image when compared to women. Do the men who circle body areas related to drugs focus more on improving (making them better through drugs) rather than coping with negative shame-filled feelings? These will be interesting dynamics to reflect back to the group for discussion.

Lead a free-flowing discussion about the circled items. Some participants may share personal stories or circumstances. Let the process unfold for 5–10 minutes.

Leader: Now look at the two cards you took from the basket that you have been keeping private. Compare the cards in your hand to the list of sex/drug-linked body image areas on the wall.

Lead a discussion about the common answers on the wall lists and the personal lists. Allow for free-flowing discussion. Some participants may share personal stories or circumstances. Let the process unfold for 5–10 minutes.

Welcome similar and dissimilar individual responses from the group. By emphasizing similar statements, you can normalize these body image concerns for men, women, or both who are in recovery. Listen for the connection between body image dissatisfaction and drug or alcohol use patterns or for attempts to improve on an already positive body part.

Leader: What are people thinking or feeling after doing this exercise?

Allow for a short debriefing discussion; welcome comments, observations, or thoughts about the experience.

Leader: We are now going to spend the remainder of the class in our separate groups for men and women.

Break into separate groups of men and women. Both groups will meet for the remainder of the session in separate rooms, each with at least one group leader.

WOMEN'S GROUP

Topic Skill Practice

Leader: We chose to spend the remainder of the class in a group for women because we know that body image issues are different for men and women. A recent study confirmed that both men and women have significant issues surrounding their relationship with their body, but the dynamics and content of the issues tend to have some distinct differences.

Who do you think generally was found to have more widespread body image concerns: men or women? Body image concerns were generally found to be more prevalent among women than men.

Who tends to be less satisfied with their bodies? Women reported lower satisfaction with their bodies.

Who tends to report concealing their bodies more frequently? Women have a greater tendency to conceal their bodies.

Who compares their appearance to that of others more frequently? Women appeared to compare their appearance to that of others more frequently than men did.

Who is more concerned about other people negatively evaluating their appearance? These gender differences tend to disappear among men and women who desire to lose weight. Men and women who want to lose weight tend to have very similar body image concerns and worries (Grogan, 2008).

Leader: A broad conceptualization of body image may prove important in understanding the nature of the construct among men. Men appear to be less inclined to hold negative attitudes toward their bodies but do report a strong motivation to improve the appearance of their bodies (Davison & McCabe, 2005). Research has found women who take part in sports have more positive perceptions of their own bodies and increased acceptance of muscular body shapes.

What all of these studies have in common is an interest in the type and amount of negative and positive body thoughts. We are calling this combination of positive and negative body thoughts your relationship with your body. Today's group will teach a specific skill to improve your relationship with your body. The skill is to become more aware of the way to think and talk to yourself about your own body.

Men and women have very different experiences with their bodies. This group will focus on specific thoughts and self-talk that you may have about your bodies. We know that for women in recovery, their personal relationship with their own body is a vital relationship for maintaining sobriety. What a woman thinks, her opinion, private comments, and criticisms, usually known only to her, can be brutally harsh, judgmental, and mean. Today's group will focus on your personal self-talk about your body. Women in recovery must stay aware of their body self-talk. Women who are unaware of negative body self-talk have a hidden risk to their sobriety. Over time, sometimes only days or weeks into recovery, a frequently negative and severe body talk will interfere with staying focused on the hard work of recovery. We are going to spend the remainder of our time together increasing your awareness of what you think and say to yourself about your body. What you think and perceive about your body will directly affect your sexual behavior in recovery.

We are going to learn body talk. Body talk is the thoughts, conversations, ideas, and typical reactions we have every day, in our own mind, our own private body self-talk. We will learn four specific types of body self-talk. Two types interfere with recovery and can lead to relapse, and two types support recovery and decrease the risk of relapse. We call these the body talk four Cs. They are:

1. Body contempt
2. Body criticism
3. Body complaint
4. Body compliment

These body talk four Cs are based on research studies by John Gottman that looked at what makes marriages work (Gottman & Silver, 1999). For better or for worse, what makes a marriage between two people work or fail may have relevance for what may make our relationship with our body, especially in recovery, be more successful. Sexual health requires a constructive and positive relationship with our body. We base our body talk four Cs on the patterns for successful and toxic ways that Dr. Gottman observed in the couples he researched.

Body contempt is self-talk that is full of sarcasm, cynicism, name-calling, sneering, and/or mockery. Body contempt self-talk is an ongoing message of disgust and hostility toward your body. It keeps you in a constant state of conflict with your body. When a women in recovery does not learn how to deal with body contempt, it leaves her in a perpetual state of conflict or even hatred with her body. Body contempt is like living with someone who is disgusted with you and lets you know how disgusted he or she is every chance he or she gets. What are examples of body contempt that we just discussed in the class?

Lead a group discussion about examples of body contempt comments. Leader may remind group of similar comments written on the note cards in the earlier full group session.

Leader: *Body criticism* is self-talk that is focused on what is wrong with your body. Body criticism looks at any specific body part or feature and finds a criticism that is stated in a big, overblown generalization.

So body criticisms will have words like "always" and "never" combined with a dash of character assassination thrown in for good measure. So it may sound a bit like: "Your stomach is so fat and ugly who is ever going to want to sleep you?" or "Your butt is so huge it's all anyone can think of when you sit down." Well, you get the picture. Dr. Gottman found in his marriage research that couples who criticized each other too frequently pointed out what was wrong with their partner in sweeping generalizations.

What are common body criticisms for women in recovery?

Facilitate a group discussion. Encourage group members to talk with each other rather than through you. Having women speak with other women about their private and lonely body hate speech is an important shame reduction component of this lesson.

Leader: The good news is that Dr. Gottman found two important ways for couples to improve their marriages, and we will teach you the same tools today. You can practice these tools for many months and years of recovery to improve your body talk and your sexual health.

The first skill is really listening to your body self-talk. Identify the conversation of body contempt and criticism you have with yourself. Knowing if you are stating a complaint about your body rather than self-hating contempt is an important body image recovery tool. Being able to accurately label a body self-talk as body contempt or body criticism is a way to begin having some influence or power over this destructive self-talk. We just did that in the group. We stepped back for a moment and labeled the body talk, gave it a name. Labeling a contemptuous statement is an important first step in reducing contempt-filled body talk. Remember, body contempt is the first harmful body conversation in our thoughts or with others to become aware of and identify.

Turning a body criticism into a *body complaint* is the second skill. A body complaint is making a statement of disappointment without judgment in regards to a specific body trait. A body complaint is a feeling of sadness because a hope or wish you have for your body is not going to happen. A body complaint is a reasonable relationship to have with our body. Just like every long-term relationship, we must learn to incorporate the disappointments that come with the complete package that also includes the parts we like. A body complaint is a more useful and nondestructive way to address aspects of your body that disappoint you. A body complaint begins with the self-talk statement:

- I am disappointed
- I am disappointed because my waist size is two inches too big for my pants.
- I am disappointed that my hair does not look as good as I want it to.
- I am disappointed that . . . (fill in the blank)

A complaint (according to Gottman) is a much more specific situation or circumstance that focuses on right now, the present. "I am very upset that my waist has grown another two inches and my pants fit me too tight." Add the words "what is wrong with you?" and you have just turned a disappointment into a more emotional and triggering criticism. Body criticism self-talk is a slow, corrosive process that can lead to body contempt. Left unattended, these forms of body self-talk can be powerful relapse triggers. They can be particularly shameful relapse triggers if you are filled with body criticism and contempt and begin to consider or experience a sexual situation or relationship. The contempt can become so intense that it can trigger thoughts and urges of using. Addressing the body contempt and criticism is a powerful tool to move toward a more enjoyable sexual life while lessoning the risk of relapse.

The last component of body image self-talk is *body compliments*. Gottman's research concluded that the balance between positive (compliments) in successful marriages and negative (contempt, criticism, and complaint) is about a 5:1 ratio. I include complaint in the negative because this was the way Gottman reviewed his data. For body image work in recovery, moving contempt and criticism into a disappointment (complaint) is significant progress for sexual health in recovery.

Gottman and Silver found the 5:1 ratio to be a reliable predictor of marital longevity. When husbands and wives expressed positive feelings with each other five times more than negative feelings the marriage was much more stable than couples with little positive to balance their increasing negativity with each other (Gottman & Silver, 1994). For men and women in recovery, the same balance is needed for a successful long-term relationship with your own body.

The "Body Self-Talk in Recovery" worksheet balances negative and positive body self-talk as a sexual health in recovery tool.

Hand out "Body Self-Talk in Recovery" worksheet.

Leader: What are the most common body contempt and body criticisms, women have about their bodies that they cope with by using drugs or alcohol? What drug(s) do women commonly use to quiet body self-talk?

Let's complete the worksheet. List a current body part/attitude that is on your mind. Check the body contempt statement that sounds most like your self-talk. Check the body criticism that sounds most like your self-talk. Check the drug that is associated with coping with this body contempt or criticism. Practice turning this into a body complaint where you give yourself permission to be disappointed without negatively or harshly judging yourself. Write five body compliments at the end.

Closing

Leader: Now let's take a moment to bring the workshop to a close. Lets take a moment to again quiet ourselves, take a deep breath to quiet our minds, our hearts, and our spirits. In this quiet place, remind yourself how valuable it is to take the time to be honest, vulnerable, and committed to recovery. As you leave the group today, remind yourself that a satisfying sexual life is a vital and important part of recovery. The self-reflection and tools you learned today may become an important part of maintaining your recovery.

MEN'S GROUP

Topic Skill Practice

Leader: We chose to spend the remainder of the class in a group for men because we know that body image issues are different for men and women. A recent study confirmed that both men and women have significant issues surrounding their relationship with their body, but the dynamics and content of the issues tend to have some distinct differences.

Who do you think generally was found to have more widespread body image concerns, men or women? Body image concerns were generally found to be more prevalent among women than men.

Who tends to be less satisfied with their bodies? Women reported lower satisfaction with their bodies.

Who tends to report concealing their bodies more frequently? Women have a greater tendency to conceal their bodies.

Who compares their appearance to that of others more frequently? Women appeared to compare their appearance to that of others more frequently than men did.

Who is more concerned about other people negatively evaluating their appearance? These gender differences tend to disappear among men and women who desire to lose weight. Men and women who want to lose weight tend to have very similar body image concerns and worries. (Grogan, 2008)

Leader: A broad conceptualization of body image may prove important in understanding the nature of the construct among men, Men appear to be less inclined to hold negative attitudes toward their bodies but do report a strong motivation to improve the appearance of their bodies (Davison & McCabe, 2005).What all of these studies have in common is an interest in the type and amount of negative and positive body thoughts. We are calling this combination of positive and negative body thoughts your relationship with your body. Today's group will teach a specific skill to improve your relationship with your body. The skill is to become more aware of the way to think and talk to yourself about your own body. Men and women have very different experiences with their bodies. This group will focus on specific thoughts and self-talk that you may have about your bodies. We know that for men in recovery, their personal relationship with their own body may be less of a preoccupation than for women in recovery.

Today's group will focus on your personal self-talk about your body. Men in recovery must stay aware of their body self-talk. Men who are unaware of negative body self-talk have a hidden risk to their sobriety. Over time, sometimes only days or weeks into recovery, a frequently negative and severe body talk will interfere with staying focused on the hard work of recovery. We are going to spend the remainder of our time together increasing your awareness of what you think and say to yourself about your body. What you think and perceive about your body will directly affect your sexual behavior in recovery.

We are going to learn body talk. Body talk is the thoughts, conversations, ideas, and typical reactions we have every day, in our own mind, our own private body self-talk. We will learn four specific types of body self-talk. Two that interfere with recovery and can lead to relapse and two that support recovery and decrease the risk of relapse. We call these the body talk four Cs. They are:

- Body contempt
- Body criticism
- Body complaint
- Body compliment

These body talk four Cs are based on research studies by John Gottman that looked at what makes marriages work (Gottman & Silver, 1999). For better or for worse, what makes a marriage between two people work or fail may have relevance for what may make our relationship with our body, especially in recovery, be more successful. Sexual health requires a constructive and positive relationship with our body. We base our body talk four Cs on the patterns for successful and toxic ways that Dr. Gottman observed in the couples he researched.

Body contempt is self-talk that is full of sarcasm, cynicism, name-calling, sneering, and mockery. Body contempt self-talk is an ongoing message of disgust and hostility toward your body. It keeps you in a constant state of conflict with your body. When a man in recovery does not learn how to deal with body contempt it leaves him in a perpetual state of conflict or even hatred with his body. Body contempt is like living with someone who is disgusted with you and lets you know how disgusted he or she is every chance he or she gets. What are examples of body contempt that we just discussed in the class?

Lead a group discussion about examples of body contempt comments. You may remind the group of similar comments written on the note cards in the earlier full group session.

Leader: *Body criticism* is self-talk that is focused on what is wrong with your body. Body criticism looks at any specific body part or feature and finds a criticism that is stated in a big, overblown generalization. So body criticisms will have words like "always" and "never" combined with a dash of character assassination thrown in for good measure. So it may sound a bit like: "Your belly is so big you'll never get laid," "I hate how short I am," or "You're loosing your hair so fast you're going to look too old for anyone to want you." Well, you get the picture. Dr. Gottman found in his marriage research that couples who criticized each other too frequently pointed out what was wrong with their partner in sweeping generalizations.

What are common body criticisms for men in recovery?

Facilitate a group discussion. Encourage group members to talk with each other rather than through you. Men speaking with other men about their private and lonely body hate speech is an important shame reduction component of this lesson.

Leader: The good news is that Dr. Gottman found two important ways for couples to improve their marriages, and we will teach you the same tools today. You can practice these tools for many months and years of recovery to improve your body talk and your sexual health. This is what Dr. Gottman found in his marriage research.

The first skill is really listening to your body self-talk. To identify the conversation of body contempt and criticism you have with yourself. Knowing if you are stating a complaint about your body rather than self-hating contempt is an important body image recovery tool. Just to accurately label body self-talk as body contempt or body criticism is a way to begin having some influence or power over this destructive self-talk. We just did that in the group. We stepped back for just a moment and labeled the body talk, gave it a name. Labeling a contemptuous statement is an important first step in reducing contempt-filled body talk. Remember, body contempt is the first harmful body conversation in our thoughts or with others to become aware of and identify.

Turning a body criticism into a *body complaint* is the second skill. A body complaint is a more useful and nondestructive way to address aspects of your body that disappoint you. A body complaint begins with the self-talk statement:

- I have a complaint . . .
- I have a complaint: my stomach is two inches too big for my pants.
- I have a complaint: I am losing my hair.
- I have a complaint: my (your fill in the blank).

A complaint (according to Gottman) is a much more specific situation or circumstance that focuses on right now, the present. "I am very upset that my waist has grown another two inches and my pants fit me too tight." Add what is wrong with you and you have just turned a specific complaint into a more emotional and triggering criticism. Body criticism self-talk is a slow, corrosive process that can lead to body contempt. Left unattended, these forms of body self-talk can be powerful relapse tools. They can be particularly shameful relapse triggers if you are filled with body criticism and contempt and begin to consider or experience a sexual situation or relationship. The contempt can become so intense that it can trigger using thoughts and urges. Addressing body contempt and criticism is a powerful tool to move toward a more enjoyable sexual life while lessoning the risk of relapse.

The last component of body image self-talk is *body compliments*. Gottman's research concluded that the balance between positive (compliments) in successful marriages and negative (contempt, criticism, and complaint) is about a 5:1 ratio. I include complaint in the negative because this was the way Gottman reviewed his data. For body image work in recovery, moving contempt and criticism into a disappointment (complaint) is significant progress for sexual health in recovery.

Gottman and Silver found the 5:1 ratio to be a reliable predictor of marital longevity. When husbands and wives expressed positive feelings with each other five times more than negative feelings the marriage was much more stable than couples with little positive to balance their increasing negativity with each other (Gottman & Silver, 1994). For men and women in recovery, the same balance is needed for a successful long-term relationship with your body.

The "Body Self-Talk in Recovery" worksheet balances negative and positive body self-talk as a sexual health in recovery tool.

Hand out the "Body Self-Talk in Recovery" worksheet (Lesson 12 appendix).

Leader: What are common body contempt, body criticism, or body complaints men have about their bodies that they cope with by using drugs or alcohol? What drug(s) do men commonly use to quiet body self-talk?

Let's complete the sheet. List a current body part/attitude that is on your mind. Check the body contempt statement that sounds most like your self-talk. Check the body criticism that sounds most like your self-talk. Check the drug that is associated with coping with this body contempt or criticism. Practice turning this into a body complaint. Write five body compliments at the end.

Closing

Leader: Now let's take a moment to bring the workshop to a close. Lets take a moment to again quiet ourselves, take a deep breath to quiet our minds, our hearts, and our spirits. In this quiet place, remind yourself how valuable it is to take the time to be honest, vulnerable, and committed to recovery. As you leave the group today, remind yourself that a satisfying sexual life is a vital and important part of recovery. The self-reflection and tools you learned today may become an important part of maintaining your recovery.

REFERENCES

Davison, T., & McCabe, M. (2005). Relationship's between men's and women's body image and their psychological, social and sexual functioning. *Journal of Sex Research,* 52(7–8), 463–475.

Foley, S., Kope, S., & Sugrue, D. (2002). *Sex matters for women: A complete guide to taking care of your sexual self.* New York: The Guilford Press.

Gottman, J. M., Gottman, J. S., & DeClaire, J. (2006). *10 Lessons to transform your marriage.* New York: Three Rivers Press.

Gottman, J., & Silver, N. (1994, March/April). What makes marriage work? Its how you resolve conflict that matters most. *Psychology Today.*

Gottman, J., & Silver, N. (1999). *The seven principles for making marriage work.* New York: Three Rivers Press.

Grogan, S. (2008). *Body image: Understanding body dissatisfaction in men, women and children* (2nd ed.). New York: Routledge.

Whitman, W. (1891). *Leaves of Grass.* Philadelphia, PA: David McKay Publisher.

LESSON 12 APPENDIX

Body Self-Talk in Recovery

This tool is designed to assist in retraining your self-commentary on your body image. For a relationship with your body to be satisfying and fulfilling, the ratio of positive to negative body statements must be about five positive statements for every negative statement. Relentless body contempt and body criticism will maintain a negative mindset that will contribute to relapse. Positive, complimentary body self-talk and honest acknowledgement of what is disappointing about your body is first-aid directly applied to the wound of body hatred. An honest complaint without harsh judgment may reduce shame-based body self-talk. Changing your body attitudes to a much more frequent positive self-talk is a practical way to prevent relapse and improve sexual health in recovery.

Directions

1. Read the list of items related to your body and your body functioning. Find an item you are noticing having negative, harsh, or punitive self-talk about today. Circle that item.

Hair	Attractiveness	Waist
How others like my body	Body build (muscles)	Height
Thighs	Breast/chest (pecs)	Eyes
Legs	Lips	Skin
Hips	Arms	Teeth
Face	Weight	Sex (male or female)
Skin color	Stomach	Penis/labia/vulva
Buttocks		

List your own (be specific):

_____

2. Is the body talk contempt or criticism? Contempt: Is the body talk demeaning? Insulting? Name calling? Mean?
3. Criticism: Always? Never? Blaming? Piling on every negative body criticism? Complaint: What am I dissatisfied with right now?

Write your complaint here:

_____

I feel dissatisfied about (list body part or feature here) today because (list the immediate situation that is happening right now):

_____

4. Is this a disappointment that I associate with using drugs/alcohol? Yes No
5. I can train myself to have a more balanced and satisfying relationship with my body. When I have body contempt or criticism I will balance this harsh judgment with five positive statements about my body:

Write your positive statements here

1. _____
2. _____
3. _____
4. _____
5. _____

Index